In memory of David Cartwright

Screening the Body

Screening the Body

Tracing Medicine's Visual Culture

Lisa Cartwright

University of Minnesota Press

Minneapolis

London

Chapter 2, " 'Experiments of Destruction': Cinematic Inscriptions of Physiology," was previously published in slightly different form in *Representations* 40 (Fall 1992); copyright 1992 by the Regents of the University of California. Reprinted by permission.

Chapter 6, "Women and the Public Culture of Radiography," was originally published as "Women, X-rays, and the Public Culture of Prophylactic Imaging," *Camera Obscura* 29 (May 1992): 18–54. Reprinted with permission of Indiana University Press.

Published by the University of Minnesota Press
111 Third Avenue South, Minneapolis, MN 55401-2520
Printed in the United States of America on acid-free paper
Second printing, 1997
Library of Congress Cataloging-in-Publication Data

Cartwright, Lisa, 1959–
   Screening the body : tracing medicine's visual culture /
Lisa Cartwright.
     p.   cm.
   Includes bibliographical references and index.
   ISBN 0-8166-2289-2
   ISBN 0-8166-2290-6 (pbk.)
   1. Motion pictures in medicine—History. 2. Medical
imaging—History.   I. Title.
   R835.C37   1995
   306.4'61–dc20   94-30340

Contents

Acknowledgments

THIS BOOK BEGAN AS A HISTORY and theory of the cinematic gaze in medical culture. Medical films are not very pretty, and it is perhaps for this reason that so little is written about them. I wanted to trace the history of the optical techniques and the moving images that set the ground for the contemporary visual analysis of the body in medicine—the field of medical imaging that has formed since midcentury into a vastly successful industry and culture. With great consternation, I found the long process of research and writing repeatedly punctuated by firsthand experiences with contemporary medical institutions and their techniques. The illnesses and deaths of family members and friends, and my own unanticipated encounters within the gynecological gaze and its new imaging technologies, constituted the most difficult and politically transformative research I did. Although the lessons that I learned firsthand during the years that I worked on this project are not a part of this book's overt content, they informed every word I wrote.

I am grateful to the following people for their help and support during my research in their archives and collections: Sarah Richards of the National Library of Medicine Historical Medical Films Collection; Michael Rhode of the National Museum of Health and Medicine; John Wandtke and Mary Lou Bryant of the University of Rochester Radiology Department; Marilyn Matz of the Library of Congress; Jan-Christopher Horak and Paolo Cherchi-Usai of the George Eastman House Film Department; Dale Davis, executor of the papers of James Sibley Watson Jr.; Christopher Hoolihan of the Miner Library, Medical History Division, at the University of Rochester; and Warren Sturges. My oldest debts are to Sander Gilman, David Rodowick, and Alan Trachtenberg for encouraging and supporting this strange project from its beginnings. For giving valuable feedback, advice, or support at different moments of this project, I thank Zelda Artson, Ali Behdad, Giuliana Bruno, Nancy Cott, Warren Crichlow, Douglas Crimp, Susan Daitch, Nina Fonoroff, Kathy Geritz, Tom Gunning, Kathy High, Serene Jones, Alex

ix

Juhasz, Caren Kaplan, Terri Kapsalis, Eric Kracauer, Audrey Kupferberg, Lev Manovich, Gregg Mitman, Constance Penley, Dana Polan, Lauren Rabinovitz, Paula Rabinowitz, Mary Renda, Fatimah Tobing Rony, Barbara Schulman, Ella Shohat, Michele Shubin, Jeff Skoller, Eric Smoodin, Vivian Sobchak, Lynn Spigel, Howard Spiro, Paula Treichler, and John Harley Warner. I am especially grateful to Paula Treichler and Constance Penley for bringing the dialogue on science, medicine, and representation into feminist film studies.

Ludmilla Jordanova's groundbreaking *Sexual Visions: Images of Gender in Science and Medicine between the Eighteenth and Twentieth Centuries* (University of Wisconsin Press, 1989) was an inspiration to me during the long process of revising my manuscript. I am indebted to the Pembroke Center for Teaching and Research on Women at Brown University for giving me a postdoctoral year in which to start that process. Thanks to Elizabeth Weed, Karen Newman, Anne Fausto-Sterling, and my comrades Leslie Camhi, Brian Cooper, and Jennifer Terry, for having terrific senses of humor and irony during our inquiry into scientific knowledge and "difference" during that year. The work of Leslie Camhi and Jenny Terry continues to be an inspiration to my own research and writing.

I am deeply indebted to my colleagues and students at Rochester for their support and inspiration. Mark Betz, Laura U. Marks, and Paul Schwankl provided valuable feedback in their meticulous proofreading and editing of the manuscript. My editor Janaki Bakhle and her assistant Robert Mosimann provided expert advice and aid.

Much of the research on which this book is based could not have been done without the support of Francesca, Henry, and Adam Barragan and Chris Sigismonti in Washington, D.C. I would never have been able to see this project through without the continual care and support of Brian Goldfarb, Francesca and Edward Perrier, Carole Goldfarb, and Ted Goldstein. My deepest debt is to Brian, who discussed and contributed to ideas and research at every stage of this book's progress.

Finally, this project would never have been started without the years of discussion, research, and activism that I shared with my late father, David Cartwright. His activist work on the legal rights of survivors of radiation testing and on the ethics of animal testing, as well as his work with people designated mentally disabled, profoundly influenced my work on this book from start to finish.

Introduction

IN THE INTRODUCTION to a recent collection of essays on the representation of women's bodies in debates about pregnancy and abortion, the historian Barbara Duden describes the emergence of the term "life" as, in her words, an idol. Duden's project takes as its starting point the familiar and dispassionate use of this term in public discourse around pregnancy, women's bodies, and obstetrics. This term leads her to consider what she describes as the graphic techniques that were used to "flay" the female body and turn it inside out to expose the body of interest—the fetus—to public view, a process that involved techniques including woodcuts, X rays, and ultrasound.[1] In this volume, I also consider the ascendancy of this term "life" as a core object of epistemological conquest in science, and the optical dissection and penetration of the human body that accompanied the popularization of this term throughout medical science, public health, and public culture generally. I have limited my project primarily to the analysis of a single, and perhaps less familiar, technology for configuring life. My object here is the cinema as an institution and an apparatus for monitoring, regulating, and ultimately building "life" in the modernist culture of Western medical science.

Michel Foucault also has discussed the emergence of something called life along with the emergence of the discipline of biology in the nineteenth century. As he points out, this historical conjuncture entailed the advancement of a new mode of representation in science.[2] This book begins with the assertion that the motion picture, in conjunction with more familiar nineteenth-century medical recording and viewing instruments and techniques, such as the kymograph, the microscope, and the X-ray apparatus, was a crucial instrument in the emergence of a distinctly modernist mode of representation in Western scientific and public culture—a mode geared to the temporal and spatial decomposition and reconfiguration of bodies as dynamic fields of action in need of regulation and control. It is a familiar claim in film scholarship that public audiences of the first motion pictures were thrilled by the sight of the body in motion. This thrill was related in important ways to the scientific techniques of analytical surveillance of bodily systems described in this volume. Popular pleasure in the sight of moving bodies was bound up with the nineteenth-century development of recording instruments and graphic techniques that afforded scientists a degree of control over bodily movement not granted through, for example, the static technique of photography. The cinema, a technology designed to record and reproduce movement, was deeply indebted to physiology, both practically and ideologically. Human physiology—the term refers both to the living body and to the science dedicated to its study—was a central force in the emergence of an instrument designed precisely to record and represent the body as a living, moving entity. As John Tagg, Sander Gilman, and Allan Sekula have shown, the static medium of photography was regarded within nineteenth-century science, medicine, and state institutions as an instrument particularly well suited to the study of anatomy and morphology.[3] Likewise, the motion picture was regarded as an apparatus uniquely suited to the study of physiology. Indeed, in the view of Terry Ramsaye, an early historian of the cinema, the motion picture apparatus actually embodied the organic laws of the life it recorded:

> He who will have the patience to follow the growth of the motion picture will find it too, like the tree, clearly an organism, following organic law in its development. The living picture will be found following that law with the unrelenting persistence that marks the growth of all living things, from yeast mold to races.
>
> It is only by this recognition of the organic character of the motion picture and its consequent interrelation to all of the organisms of mankind and society that it can be truly understood. Critics and forecasters, academic, professional, and commercial, are continually committing themselves to error, and to the swift exposure of these errors, because of their failure to see the screen as one of those strands of the yarn of life, with an affinity beyond and ahead.[4]

For Ramsaye, the cinema followed the developmental laws of Western science—"organic" laws that dictated not only the growth of trees but also the evolution of "races." Ramsaye's claim that the cinema is an organic being is clearly more than metaphorical. His comparison of the organic growth of the cinema to on the one hand yeast mold and on the other "races" demonstrates the degree to which the technology had become imbricated in naturalized cultural schemes of development and social order. In this passage we find evidence of the belief that, in the early twentieth century, a cultural technology like the cinema could be seen as an actual instance of the very laws of nature that science and medicine sought to expose to view. The descriptions of life as a complex network or system of which we find examples throughout nineteenth- and twentieth-century culture demonstrate that in fields such as

biology and physiology nature and technology were set forth as interconsti-
tutive forces in the social management of bodies, a project that can be traced
to the life-controlling and life-generating agendas of fields like genetics and
biomedicine.

The chapters of this book take up historical instances of the use of the cinema in medical science to analyze, regulate, and reconfigure the transient,
uncontrollable field of the body. Foucault has described the penetration of
the medical gaze into the interior of the body in the practice of pathological
anatomy as "the technique of the corpse."[5] He notes that the opening up of
the body in autopsy in hopes of exposing to sight the seat of disease ultimately failed to render pathology fully visible but led the physician instead to
traces of the disease mapped upon organs and surfaces. The qualitative and
empirical gaze of eighteenth- and early-nineteenth-century anatomoclinical
perception that Foucault describes overlapped with and was ultimately challenged by the relentlessly analytical and quantitative gaze demonstrated in
the cases considered in this volume, a mode of perception carefully incu-
bated within the laboratories of physiologists and medical scientists and finding its expression in an unlikely range and mix of institutions and practices,
including the hospital, the popular cinema film, the scientific experiment,
and the modernist artwork.

The following chapters trace the course of this vivifying physiological gaze
through the technologies and the bodies of living subjects. This course is
considered not chronologically but conceptually. I consider the ways that
the cinema was used as a technique to rejuvenate pathological anatomy's object of study, the corpse, rendering life an elusive and seductive object of scientific conquest. Chapter 1 makes a case for a rereading of the cinema's
history and theory through its intersections with the field of physiology. In
chapter 2, I consider the cultural implications of physiology's analytical gaze
and the relation of the body and technology put forth in the early scientific
cinema. The films of early-twentieth-century physiologists working in biology, zoology, neurology, and bacteriology constitute a critical but unconsidered moment in the history of early scientific cinema. I submit these films as
evidence that, at the turn of the century, the motion picture apparatus was
crucial in the emergence of a new set of optical techniques for social regulation. In laboratory culture, medical practice, and beyond, we see the emergence of a distinctly suveillant cinema.

In chapter 3, I begin by considering the photographic motion studies of
the chemist Albert Londe, who worked as chief photographer under the
neurologist Jean-Martin Charcot at the Paris Salpêtrière asylum. At issue
here are the practice of imaging involuntary movement and the inscription
of cultural meaning upon that familiar field of signification, the epidermis. I
discuss how the meanings affixed to the bodily surface change with the shift-

ing status of visuality in scientific knowledge after Charcot's time. Two groups of neurological films are the main focus of this chapter, each representing a distinct moment in the history of the neurological film motion study after Charcot. I argue that as vision proves itself incapable of providing neurologists with knowledge about the etiology of mental diseases, the image increasingly becomes the site of a certain professional anxiety. The neurological image finally can be seen as an inscription of the failure of neurologists to gain access to knowledge of the bodies that populate their field. The neurological film motion study, I argue, is an image of patients' agency insofar as the bodies they depict resist the meanings imposed upon them by medicine. But these films are also the symbolic embodiment of neurology's own failed powers of vision over the bodies it seeks to manage.

In chapter 4, I consider the ways in which the technique of microscopic cinematography has been used to analyze the minute and interior systems of the body during the same years in which neurology scrutinized the body's surface. Here I pursue the argument that twentieth-century medicine does not so much "flay" the body as it does away with distinctions of interior/exterior or object/ground. Further, the body is rendered part of a living system that incorporates the technologies of its representation. I consider the intersections between microscopy's modes of representation and conventions in modernist art, using cubism as my specific example. A secondary theme of this chapter is the relationship between modernist science and modernist art and film movements. My thesis is not merely that the two areas were mutually constitutive, but that conventions of visuality in techniques of knowledge and power emerge across disparate and apparently unrelated cultures and contexts, and thus it is necessary to consider the extent that modernist art and modernist science are mutually implicated in the emergence of modern biomedicine and its particular techniques of analyzing and refabricating "life."

Chapter 5 extends the analysis of the visual decomposition of the body begun in chapter 3 to an extended consideration of the techniques of X ray and X-ray cinematography. Here I begin with the premise that medical techniques have, from their origins, been informed by popular and subcultural views of the body. My analysis of X-ray cinema also allows me to consider more closely the place of death, life, and pleasure in the medical gaze, and the fate of the profilmic body in this conjuncture. Whereas chapter 4 focuses on the construction of a film body that is celebrated for its aliveness, chapter 5 uncovers the historical construction of a body that is feared and revered for its evocation of death in life. The X-ray motion picture that apparently "flays" the body for observation is ultimately a caricature and travesty of the scientific obsession with "life."

The analysis of X rays presented in chapter 5, as in the previous chapters, focuses primarily on knowledge, pleasure, and desire in the relatively private space of the laboratory. In these chapters I provide very little analysis of, for example, the popular reception of microscopy, the enthusiastic reception of science motion studies in public theaters, or even the dissemination of the techniques I describe into clinics and hospitals. In the final chapter, I consider the role of public culture in the institutionalization of the X ray as the primary medical imaging technology of this century. Here I consider specifically the work of women patients, technologists, and community members in the operation of radiography's disciplining gaze. My focus is the public media campaign against tuberculosis at midcentury (a campaign that included the mass institution of the chest X ray as a TB screening technique) and the later campaign to institute and popularize mass X-ray screening for breast cancer. Earlier chapters of this book can perhaps be faulted for taking to an extreme the thesis that the cinema was used in science as a strategy of control and domination. This final chapter, then, is an attempt to rework the material covered in chapter 5 in order to uncover a subjugated history of those individuals and communities who were the objects of the surveillant and analytical medical gaze. Here I tell a less totalizingly condemning story of scientific visuality, one that acknowledges the benefits and possibilities of medical imaging, and one that acknowledges more fully the diverse cultures and identities implicated in medical culture. Although this chapter in some ways breaks both thematically and methodologically with earlier ones, I have allowed these differences to stand, rather than attempting to recast earlier arguments.

It is important to say a word about my process in selecting material from among the vast quantity of medical and scientific films and writings I unearthed in researching this project. I spent two years viewing the film holdings and digging through the archives of such institutions as the National Library of Medicine, the National Museum of Health and Medicine, the Library of Congress, and the National Archives. I also visited private collections in homes and hospitals. There were many films that I viewed but for a variety of reasons finally chose not to discuss. Some films I omitted because they were so clearly beyond the scope of legitimate medical practice. In this category, for example, are the films of a New York Beth Israel Hospital gynecologist who filmed women patients while subjecting them to experimental vaginal electroshock "therapy." Unlike the radiology experiments described in chapter 5, this project fit no broader pattern of film practice and was so blatantly an instance of exploitation without medical justification that it didn't merit discussion. Other films not discussed here certainly do deserve analysis but were ultimately outside the scope of my project. A category of film that fits this description is the more conventional documentary medical film—for example, those didactic films that were produced primarily to be shown as teaching demonstrations, rather than as experimental studies (demonstrations of surgical techniques, for example). My decision was to focus on research films produced in the process of analyzing a disease or condition, and to work my way through the modernist logic of abstraction and analysis that informed the more mundane and obscure nonrepresentational films that seemed to me to be so clearly linked to the "new" imaging technologies that we find in hospitals and clinics today. Therefore I left out many important instances in the history of the medical film. However, there is certainly an essay to be written about the notorious Doctor Doyen, the surgeon whose "teaching films" doubled as public entertainment spectacles in turn-of-the-century France. Also deserving of future consideration is the popular reception of microscopic films—for example, Percy Smith's macroscopic and microscopic films that were so enthusiastically received in England in the early decades of this century. Worth noting too are the obstetrical teaching films of Joseph B. DeLee, medical school teaching texts that graphically demonstrate the outrageous beliefs and practices of the U.S. obstetrical and gynecological community at midcentury. These films would be particularly useful points of reference in discussions of contemporary imaging techniques in obstetrics.

Two chapters that were in fact written but finally did not make it into this volume consider the cinematic time and motion studies of Frank Gilbreth (which deal primarily with movement in the industrial workplace but also briefly consider the movement of the surgeon's hand) and the prolific film production unit of the Army Medical Museum during World War I, a body of work that includes a substantial number of time and motion study films influenced directly by the work of Marey and Muybridge. Although I conducted extensive archival research on many of these subjects, they ultimately fell outside the scope of this project. As will be clear throughout this volume, my intention was not to provide an exhaustive historical record of the medical motion picture but to consider the status of visuality in knowledge about and authority over the body, gender, and cultural identity in medical science in the first half of this century. It is my hope that this account may inform and contribute to the study of contemporary medical imaging and the multivalent forms of contemporary visual culture. For a detailed history of the medical film, I direct readers to a very informative (but unfortunately unpublished) circa-1950 manuscript by Adolf Nichtenhauser, which is housed in the National Library of Medicine.[6] This manuscript provides a thorough narrative account of European and North American medical film that is lacking in my study; and a 1955 book by Anthony Michaelis provides a more technical and theoretical account of the medical research film.[7] Michaelis's study demonstrates my case throughout this volume about the scientific designation of movement as a prime characteristic of life and frame analysis as the key to scientific knowledge about life. Michaelis's book is also notable for its chapter on motion study in anthropology, a subject analyzed at length by Fatimah Tobing Rony.[8]

I approach my topic not as a historian of science but as a scholar of U.S. media and visual culture. This book purports to be neither an exhaustive historical narrative of the science film as a documentary subgenre nor an account of the cinema's technological history. It is a close analysis of particular moments and techniques in the history of a largely unexamined field of visual culture, that of medical and scientific imaging. This volume, though it is a close reading of texts and technologies, reveals some of the ways in which scientific knowledge and scientific subjectivities are resolutely entangled with a broad range and mix of cultural and representational practices, and thus cannot be adequately understood from within a single disciplinary framework or a single national context. How, for example, could I have limited my discussion of the decorative X rays of women's bejeweled hands and bodies (described in chapters 5 and 6) to an analysis of scientific discourse alone, when these images so clearly served as popular icons in public culture? And what can be said about a national science or a national cinema in the case of the neurological films (discussed in chapter 3) produced by German neurologists after their emigration to the United States—scientists trained in German medicine during the 1930s but claiming a status within a transnational discourse across nothing less than "the world of science"? The purpose of this study, then, is not only to fill in gaps in the canons of film studies and the social studies of science, but also to demonstrate how the cinema, an instrument of popular entertainment, functioned as a part of a social apparatus through which the cultures of Western science and medicine shaped and built the life they studied, and how individual subjects and cultures aided, confounded, or resisted Western medical science's normative life-building projects in the first half of this century.

CHAPTER 1

Science and the Cinema

IN THE BIOGRAPHICAL FILES of the New York Academy of Medicine, sharing a page with news entries documenting French claims to international railway speed and air flight records, appears a 1954 obituary for Auguste Lumière, patriarch of the cinema.[1] The appearance of Lumière's obituary among these items is not surprising. The Cinématographe, an instrument for the recording and projection of living motion invented by Lumière and his brother Louis in 1895, certainly would seem to deserve a place alongside these technologies of movement.[2] However, the obituarist barely notes Lumière's reputation as a founder of the cinema. Instead, he extols his near-lifelong commitment to medical biology, pharmacology, and experimental physiology.

After 1900 Lumière's work, and much of the production of the Lumière plant in Lyons, turned toward medical research and production. The obituarist singles out as Lumière's most significant accomplishment not his work on the cinema but his laboratory research on tuberculosis and cancer, diseases that continue to elude scientific control even now, at the end of the twentieth century. By the end of his life, Lumière believed scientific medical research to be one of the most important areas of work in Western culture. In a text on the achievements of science published six years before his death, he attributes Western progress to advances in pharmaceutical and medical technology:

> It would be impossible to deny that the discoveries of Science always have affected Humanity's material progress. . . . Formal proof of this is found in the fact that these discoveries have permitted the existence of man to be prolonged to the point that the average life span has tripled since the beginning of our century.[3]

Although he here cites the prolonged life span as proof of "Humanity's material progress," Lumière relegates the Cinématographe, an instrument of mass culture that can record but does not appear to alter the body physically, *1* to a few anecdotal pages near the close of the book.[4] Oddly, Lumière does not explain that many of his European and North American contemporaries regarded his popular invention as a key contribution to physiology—the very field of research through which he contributed to the advancement of French public health and the prolongation of the average life span. Certainly he was not unaware of the use of his invention in physiological research. In addition to the manufacture of products for a mass-audience cinema, the Lumière laboratory designed and produced specialized cameras and film stock for the laboratories of scientists and physicians—researchers for whom the Cinématographe was no less an instrument of physiological research than the microscope or the kymograph (a rotating drum-shaped apparatus used to inscribe movement in a wavelike linear trace).[5]

Lumière's historical elision of his own popular invention from the history of science and medicine is symptomatic of a broader disregard for the cultural implications of the technological interdependency of science and forms of popular culture. It is a commonplace of film scholarship that the popularization of the serial motion photography of physiological movement produced by Etienne-Jules Marey in France and Eadweard Muybridge in the United States was key to the technological development of the cinema,[6] and a few early film histories describe the scientific film as an important genre of the early cinema.[7] However, what remains largely unconsidered is the extent to which the particular visual modes that were operative in laboratory techniques like kymography and chronophotography, or in the science film, are integral to other genres of the cinema and of popular visual culture.

Scholarly descriptions of many Lumière films as realist do underscore their indebtedness to the genre of the science film. Lumière films such as *La sortie des usines Lumière à Lyon* (1895) or *Arrivée d'un train en gare de Villefranche-sur-Saône* (1895) are cited often as precursors of documentary cinema. Alan Williams suggests that actuality films like these were implicated in the popular science genre of the 1890s media and press. His point is that the Lumière public "was presumed to be interested in the question of the 'realism' of the images, though certainly *not for the sake of the subjects represented* but for the demonstration they afforded of 'scientific' interest and technical virtuosity."[8] Williams implies that these films qualified as realist because they allowed living movement to be observed, and not because they depicted "real" events. "What was documented," he explains, "was the work of the apparatus itself."[9]

In this book, I examine closely the place of film in the scientific project of observing the movement of living bodies, in order to propose an alternative to the designation of the science film as a documentary and realist mode of representation. I suggest that the scientific analyses of living bodies conducted in laboratories of medicine and science were in fact based in a tradition that broke with the photographic and theatrical conventions that would inform both the documentary and the narrative cinema—a tradition that is linked to laboratory instruments of graphic inscription and measurement such as the myograph, the kymograph, and the electrocardiograph. Scientific interest in physiological movement and its technological instrumentation is indebted precisely to the modes and techniques of motion recording and observation developed by experimental physiologists in France and Germany throughout the nineteenth century, those physiologists whose work falls within Auguste Lumière's "other" field, medical science.

One of my primary claims here is that the cinematic apparatus can be considered as a cultural technology for the discipline and management of the human body, and that the long history of bodily analysis and surveillance in medicine and science is critically tied to the history of the development of the cinema as a popular cultural institution and a technological apparatus. Accounts of the prehistory of the cinema almost always begin with a description of the legacy of science in the cinema vis-à-vis the physiological motion studies of Muybridge and Marey. It is by now a commonplace of film history that many of the techniques and instruments that contributed to the emergence of the cinema were designed and used by scientists, and that they were developed as a means of investigation into optics and physiology. As F. A. Talbot, the author of a 1912 history of the motion picture, explains,

> In its very earliest stages the value of animated photography was conceded to be in the field of science rather than that of amusement. [Marey] realized the inestimable value of "chronophotography" for the study and investigation of moving bodies, the rapidity in the changes of the position or form of which was impossible to follow otherwise.[10]

The historical narrative quickly shifts, however, from science to popular culture. Marey, the story goes, by failing to see the value of the Cinématographe, failed to bring the film motion study into the twentieth century. His rejection of the Cinématographe, an instrument so heavily laden with the promise of visual technology's future, coincides with the moment of the birth of the cinema in the public sphere, its availability to mass audiences in public screening halls. The prehistory of the cinema is conventionally told as a tale of early scientific experimentation marked by a break with science around 1895 with the emergence of a popular film culture and industry.

What this narrative leaves out is that the scientific film culture that contributed to the emergence of the popular cinema thrived beyond 1895, extending well into the twentieth century. This book traces the course of scientific cinema into the twentieth century, a history elided from most film history texts. But my aim here is not simply to set the film historical record straight. The history of the cinematic motion study is a crucial part of the history of the human body. Through such techniques as cinematic motion study, the body was measured, regulated, and reconceptualized in medicine and science. My aim then is to trace the history of this reconfiguration of the body through scientific techniques of motion recording and analysis—techniques that were used to put forth a model of the body as a dynamic, distinctly living and moving, system. A history of the film motion study is thus also a part of the history of twentieth-century scientific knowledge and power. This volume seeks to uncover a history of the cinematic techniques that science has used to control, discipline, and construct the human body as a technological network of dynamic systems and forces. But it also seeks to demonstrate that this history is complexly interwoven with other areas of visual culture.

I argue throughout this book that the importance of the film motion study is primarily neither its contribution to a singular dominant industry or optical paradigm nor its contribution to medical knowledge. Its greatest importance is its function as an intertext between popular and professional representations of the body as the site of human life and subjectivity. As a mode of knowledge, the film motion study is interesting less for what it showed researchers about the mechanics of human life than for what it tells us now about the cultural desires, pleasures, and fantasies surrounding the modernist dynamic model of "life" generated in physiology and medical science and advanced through technologies like the cinema. The film body of the motion study thus is a symptomatic site, a region invested with fantasies about what constituted "life" for scientists and the lay public in the early twentieth century, and anxieties about whether the "life" scientists studied in the laboratory was something that could be seen, imaged, and ultimately controlled (whether by prolonging it, as Lumière wished to do, or by having the authority to determine the moment of death).

Throughout this book, I consider instances in science in which film is implicated in the task of tracing the movements and changes of the body's systems and processes. I argue that, on one level, this cinematic tracking of the human body was a form of medical surveillance and social control. In this sense, the films I consider can be seen as a counterpart to the institutional practice of using photography to classify, to diagnose, and to maintain control over subjects deemed criminal, mentally ill, or otherwise aberrant.[11] But I also show that these films contributed to the generation of a broad cultural definition of the body as a characteristically dynamic entity—one uniquely suited to motion recording technologies like the cinema, but also one peculiarly unsuited to static photographic observation because of its changeability and interiority. Many of the films described in this volume were the culmination of years of effort on the part of scientists to glimpse a view of the body's interior systems in action. But, as I will try to show, this compulsion to reveal the interior technologies of the living body on motion-picture film involved a break with older conventions of photography and, perhaps paradoxically, instituted a crisis in scientific observation generally. The cinema I trace in the following chapters, then, is a cinema that is linked in important ways not only to the traditions of photography and the theater but also to a nonpictorial system of representation functioning in science throughout the nineteenth century, a tradition that emerged with physiology, the science devoted to the study of living systems in motion.

In the section that follows, I attempt to theorize this nonpictorial tradition of cinematic representation through accounts of the cinematic apparatus in order to ground my discussion of this distinctly nonpictorial, analytic, and surveillant cinema. My intention is to show that theories of the apparatus and spectatorship have not adequately accounted for the long-term impact of the scientific culture and economy so prevalent in the cinema's early history. Moreover, the techniques of scientific observation and analysis considered throughout this volume constitute a mode of visuality that subtends some popular cinema genres in subtle but important ways. The pleasures of "distanced" analytic viewing, I argue, are not peculiar to the genre of the motion study but have pervaded the popular cinema and other institutions. Surveillant looking and physiological analysis, then, are not just techniques of science. They are broadly practiced techniques of everyday public culture.

A Scientific Cinematic Apparatus

Theories of the cinematic apparatus, centering on the writings of Christian Metz and Jean-Louis Baudry in the late 1960s and Jean-Louis Comolli in the early 1970s, opened up a space for the consideration of the cinema as a cultural technology. In summarizing this vein of film theory in 1978, Stephen Heath emphasizes the grounding of the concept of the apparatus in the historical framework of ideology. He thus distinguishes the approach to the subject informed by Marxism, psychoanalysis, and semiotics from the technological determinism that characterized the majority of previous historiographical accounts of cinematic technology.[12] Heath takes as his example a program announcement for the historic Lumière screening at the Grand Café in 1895, a document that highlights cinematic technology at the expense of a description of the actual films whose showing it announces. Heath uses the term "machine interest" to characterize the overriding public attention to the cinema's instrumentation apparent in this announcement:

> In the first moments of the history of the cinema, it is the technology which provides the immediate interest: what is promoted and sold is the experience of the machine, the apparatus.[13]

Heath suggests, like Williams, that this moment in cinema's history is marked by a fascination with the technology of movement rather than with the image itself. But with the rise of film narrative, interest in the complexities of content would soon surpass this simple fascination with the technology of movement. Heath suggests that Baudry, Metz, and Comolli, like the early film spectator, were also captivated with the technological apparatus when they theorized the cinema in their pivotal essays on the cinematic apparatus:

> As though returning to something of those first moments, theoretical work today has increasingly been directed towards posing the terms of the "cinema-machine," the "basic apparatus," the "institution" of cinema, where "cinema" is taken more widely than the habitual notion of the cinema industry to include the "interior machine" of the psychology of the spectator.[14]

Among these theorists, Comolli goes farthest toward acknowledging the place of the economic and ideological within the cinema's technological history.[15] However, he establishes a relation between technology and the social in a hierarchical chronology that effectively separates the technical from its post-1895 social context. Comolli argues that technical components of the cinema (camera, projector, a "strip of images") were "already there, more or less invented, a long time before the formal invention of the cinema." With this prehistoric set of instruments in place, "the cinema is born immediately as a social machine" in 1895 with verification of its profitability as public spectacle.[16] Comolli further asserts, "One could just as well propose that it is the spectators who invent cinema."[17] Comolli privileges the role of public exhibition in his account of the cinematic apparatus. But how do we account for the epistemological and ideological baggage brought to the public cinema of 1895 through the "prehistoric" set of instruments "already there" at its origins? Or, to put this question another way, what techniques of power and knowledge were carried into the post-1895 popular cinema from the laboratories of our cinematic patriarchs (the Lumières, Edison, and Marey, for example)?

In his critique of myths of cinema origins, Comolli relies on the historian Jacques Deslandes to support his main argument that the cinema is finally determined not by disinterested science but by a commercial profit motive.[18] Questioning technological-determinist accounts that trace the cinema's history through a series of inventions and technologies that culminate in the public exhibitions of 1895, Comolli ultimately reasserts this date as a moment of last-instance economic determination. Interpreting the dictum that "a machine is always social before it is technical" as a chronological scheme, Comolli views cinema technology after 1895 through the logic of this social moment. Its instruments and techniques "already there, more or less ready," the prehistory of the cinema is historically situated according to a singular future mark: The "hundreds of little machines . . . destined for a more or less clumsy reproduction of the image and the movement of life" wait for the factor of exhibition, on which hinges the status of the cinema machine as a social technology.[19]

Comolli makes a crucial historical oversight in dismissing the "hundreds of little machines" of the nineteenth century as props predestined for an end-of-century mass "frenzy of the visible." As Comolli himself has emphasized, cinema's prehistory is rife with inconsistencies, "blanks and gaps."[20] Yet there is an order and economy to this "prehistoric" field. Many of these machines, the numerous cameras, projectors, and compound instruments that emerged over the course of the nineteenth century, in fact were no mere little machines, the silly contraptions of amateur inventors; they were fairly sophisticated instruments used in laboratories of physics, chemistry, and physiology. Understanding the social context of the laboratory—its technology, its economy, its own cultural modes of spectatorship—is no simple matter of evoking an unspecified artisanal science or a generalized technology. The cinema's emergence cannot be properly conceived without acknowledging the fascination with visibility that marked the preceding decades of nineteenth-century Western science.

Heath's emphatically uttered list, *"camera, movement, projection, screen,"*[21] hints at the complex sliding between the psychological and the technological in theories of the cinematic apparatus. The terms signify mechanical aspects of the cinema while also evoking one of Freud's models for psychical processes. Baudry quotes Freud's comparison of the psyche to the instruments of photography or microscopy as indication of "an optical construct which signals term for term the cinematographic apparatus." The passage from Freud is as follows:

> What is presented to us in these words is the idea of a psychical locality. I shall entirely disregard the fact that the mental apparatus with which we are concerned is also known to us in the form of an anatomical preparation, and I shall carefully avoid the temptation to determine psychical locality in an anatomical fashion. I shall remain upon psychological ground, and I propose simply to follow the suggestion that we should picture the instrument which carries out our mental functions as resembling a compound microscope or a photographic apparatus, or something of the kind. On that basis, psychical locality will correspond to a point inside the apparatus at which one of the preliminary stages of an image comes into being. In the microscope and telescope, as we know, these occur in parts at ideal points, regions in which no tangible component to the apparatus is situated.[22]

Baudry justifies Freud's later exclusion of the camera from this model, and his turn to the telescope or microscope, by claiming that "the cinema is already too technologically determined an apparatus for describing the psychical apparatus as a whole." He then insists that the cinema and the Neoplatonic ocular subject it constructs should have remained an important reference point for Freud's historical subject. However, putting aside the fact that the compound microscope and the telescope were also highly overdetermined instruments at the time of Freud's writing, it remains that the camera, the microscope, and the telescope offer not one but three distinct optical models for a psychical apparatus. With their respective bases in representational structures very different from the pictorial and perspectival tradition on which the camera is based, the microscope and the telescope create some problems in Baudry's theory.

Baudry's rereading of the scene of Plato's cave privileges the cinema projector and not the camera. The use of firelight evokes the artificial light source within the projector. Shadow-images suggest the perspectival film image on the screen. The trancelike state of the cave occupants is linked to the passive state of the film viewer, not the mobile and controlling gaze of the cinematographer. In Baudry's account, the womblike cave becomes the site an intermediary lens, a "point inside the apparatus at which one of the preliminary stages of an image comes into being." The subject is thus incorporated within the apparatus as a passive spectator.

As Joan Copjec has argued, theories of the cinematic apparatus present the cinema as an instrument of totalizing social control—a theoretical fantasy that is at bottom a "delirium of clinical perfection."[23] But what happens to Baudry's model if the camera is replaced with a different optical instrument—the compound microscope, for example, an instrument that the Lumières used in conjunction with the camera?[24] The compound microscope contains not one but two lenses, an interior lens for magnification and a second for resolution. The microscope offers neither empirical nor interior view for comparison. The minute object viewed through it is not available to sight by eye; likewise, the magnified image on the interior lens is unresolved and therefore not empirically visible. The spectator incorporated within this apparatus would be implicated uncomfortably in the resolution of a rather startling and unfamiliar scene, a scene that must be made sense of, or resolved, without a profilmic, or promicroscopic, referent. The microscopic spectator would be compelled to perform a very different operation inside the apparatus, one that would involve a kind of interpretive analysis that would position the spectator in a much less secure relation to visual knowledge than Baudry's model of the filmic spectator suggests.

These speculations on the possibilities of a microscopic spectator in Plato's cave are put forth simply to demonstrate that the scientific cinema, its technical spectator, and its filmed bodies make up an aspect of the cinematic apparatus that breaks in crucial ways with paradigms of cinematic technology and spectatorship generated in film scholarship around narrative and pictorial film texts and genres. I would argue that medical and scientific film motion studies provide evidence of a mode of cinematic representation and spectatorship that is grounded in a Western scientific tradition of surveillance, measurement, and physical transformation through observation and analysis. The films I study in this volume provide one of the few routes to re-historicizing the cinema as an apparatus that historically has taken place in the emergence of Lumière's fantasmatic construction of "human life" as a dynamic entity to be tracked, studied, and transformed in the social "theater" of the laboratory.

The "Frenzy of the Visible" in the Cinema's Prehistory

In a study on the relationship between science and the arts, the historian Jacob Opper suggests that changes in theories of nature from the eighteenth to the nineteenth century are best characterized by the shift from the logico-mathematical cosmology of the Enlightenment to the Darwinian biologico-evolutionary model. The example of the German physicist Ernst Mach's "phenomenological physics" is cited to convey the move toward empirical, body-based models even within the physical sciences. Opper summarizes:

> The conspicuous feature of the change in theory of nature from the eighteenth to the nineteenth centuries is thus seen to involve a shift from mathematical physics to natural-history biology, from the noumenon to the phenomenon, from the " 'logocentrism' of traditional epistemology" to " 'biocentrically oriented' romantic thought."[25]

Opper suggests that this biocentric orientation characterizes Western cultural production through the nineteenth century, the metaphor of the living, evolving organism replacing the metaphor of the mechanical, nonevolving clock.

Foucault also remarks on the nonexistence of biology prior to the nineteenth century. However, he makes a critical distinction between natural history and biology, a distinction that has important implications for his descriptions of a scientific and medical gaze and, subsequently, for the cinema as a technology of medical and scientific representation by the late nineteenth century:

> Historians want to write histories of biology in the eighteenth century; but they do not realize that biology did not exist then, and that this pattern of knowledge that has been familiar to us for a hundred and fifty years is not valid for a previous period. And that, if biology was unknown, there was a very simple reason for it: that life itself did not exist. All that existed was living beings, which were viewed through a grid of knowledge constituted by natural history.[26]

In quoting Foucault I want to emphasize that the shift from natural history to biology entailed a shift in modes of visuality, and that with the emergence of a mode of representation specific to biology, we find the emergence of "life" as a cultural concept. Foucault states that the shift from eighteenth-century natural history to nineteenth-century biology is marked by a change in relationship between representations and things. The emergence of "life" thus is accompanied by the emergence of a new mode of representation. By the time of Lamarck, the "grid of knowledge," the table of representations through which living beings had been viewed, would no longer provide a foundation for Western thought:

> The space of order, which served as a *common place* for representations and for things, for empirical visibility and for the essential rules . . . which displayed the empirical sequence of representations in a simultaneous table, and made it possible to scan step by step, in accordance with a logical sequence, the totality of nature's elements thus rendered contemporaneous with one another—this space of order is from now on shattered: there will be things, with their own organic structures, their hidden veins, the space that articulates them, the time that produces them; and then representations, a purely temporal succession, in which those things address themselves (always partially) to a subjectivity, a consciousness, a singular effort of cognition, to the "psychological" individual who from the depth of his own history . . . is trying to know. Representation is in the process of losing its power to define the mode of being common to things and to knowledge.[27]

Foucault suggests that biological representation no longer defines living beings descriptively but functions according to a structure that language cannot fully describe. This structure is "the dark, concave, inner side" of the visibility of things/living beings.[28] Whereas the grid of natural history brought living beings to full knowledge, biological representation seeks to get at what cannot be seen in a process that makes all the more evident the disjuncture between representation and "object" (or body). This formulation is far from the ideal of a romantic naturalism suggested in Opper's combined term "natural-history biology," by which nature, in direct correspondence with its science, serves as model for cultural form. It is even farther from both the space of the spectatorial cave and the pictorial space of Renaissance painting that Baudry suggests as models for cinematographic space. With the emergence of biological modes of representation, we find a historical break between observation (or image) and object of knowledge—a break in which the visualization of "life" becomes all the more seductive to the scientific eye even as the limitations of representation are made plain.

The medical gaze Foucault describes is dependent on a history of empirical techniques of diagnosis or investigation—palpation and auscultation are precedents to the empirical investigation by sight of the body's interior surfaces in the process of autopsy. Palpation and observation are marked by a temporal immediacy: on one level, diagnosis takes the form of direct contact between the physician's eye, ear, or hand with the patient's body; on another level, disease is understood to leave a visible imprint on surface tissue, in a superimposing or mapping process. In Foucault's account, even when the symptom is empirically seen, it is regarded as an indicator of a pathological condition at a different anatomical site. Paradoxically, as imaging becomes a more central means of diagnosis and study throughout the nineteenth century, sensory perception (including sight) is progressively destabilized as a source of anatomical knowledge.

It is important that the gaze Foucault identifies is tied to clinical, and not laboratory, medicine. The medical historian Robert G. Frank Jr. points out that postrevolution France saw the development not only of clinical medicine but of pathology and physiology in laboratory medical research.[29] Experimental physiology gained institutional prominence in early–nineteenth-century Germany through the laboratory research of figures such as Hermann von Helmholtz, Karl Ludwig, and Rudolph Virchow and their students. In France, physiology advanced as a specialized area of medical research in part distinct from the clinical sphere through the work of figures such as Marie-François-Xavier Bichat, Charles Edouard Brown-Séquard, and Claude Bernard. Bichat performed as a clinician; Bernard did not. This distinction is important in establishing methodological differences between practices confined to experimentation and those with more direct ties to the public sphere. Thus, the "chemical gaze" Foucault describes, while not precisely that of the laboratory scientist alone, is not wholly congruent with the clinician's gaze.

A second and more crucial distinction must be noted. Although pathological anatomy, the area of Foucault's concern, centered its representations more closely on a static concept of morphology and structure, physiology— the discipline for which the film motion study was a crucial technique—regarded the body in terms of its living functions and processes, and its practitioners devised methods and techniques to facilitate a temporal, dynamic vision of the body in motion. While this progression from stasis to movement, from anatomy to physiology, seems to suggest a narrative of technological advance, it must be kept in mind that physiology did not replace anatomy but emerged as a related specialization in its own right. The continual exchange between these fields, like the interchange between photography and the cinema, informed the filmic elaboration of life as an entity that was both temporally and spatially constituted in modernist science.

In separate studies, the medical historians Merriley Borell and Stanley Reiser have shown that the institution of physiology as a medical discipline coincided with the development of mechanical techniques and instruments for the graphic registration of bodily processes.[30] Well in advance of the development of cinematography, and independently from photography, physiologists developed visual instruments to gauge the course of normal and pathological processes qualitatively.[31] During the decades before 1895, a highly sophisticated method of graphic visual representation took shape through German and French physiology. The use of photography for physiognomical measurement is well documented in the writings of Sander Gilman, Alan Sekula, and John Tagg.[32] Tagg, in his account of the use of photography in nineteenth-century public institutions, summarizes concisely the argument that photography functioned as a representational strategy of corporeal control:

> We are dealing with the instrumental deployment of photography in privileged administrative practices and the professionalised discourses of the new social sciences—anthropology, criminology, medical anatomy, psychiatry, public health, urban planning, sanitation, and so on, all of them domains of expertise in which arguments and evidence were addressed to qualified peers and circulated only in certain limited institutional discourses. . . . In terms of such discourses, the working classes, colonized peoples, the criminal, poor, ill-housed, sick or insane were constituted as the passive—or, in this structure, "feminised"—objects of knowledge. Subjected to a scrutinizing gaze, forced to emit signs, yet cut off from command of meaning, such groups were represented as, and wishfully rendered, incapable of speaking, acting, or organizing for themselves. The rhetoric of photographic documentation at this period . . . is therefore one of precision, measurement, calculation, and proof.[33]

Tagg's description can also be applied to the cinematic practices that are described throughout this book. But it is important to note that these films, as well as the photographic practices Tagg describes, supplemented a range of more commonly used scopes, recording devices, and measurement instruments in nineteenth-century institutions. Instruments like the sphygmoscope (a device for rendering the pulse visible), the myograph (an apparatus for recording muscular contractions), and the cardiograph (an instrument for tracing the heartbeat) were as crucial as photographic analysis to the scientific disciplining of bodies and communities. The technique of cinematography, however, was paradoxically grounded in a tradition of inscription that eschewed the visual and pictorial conventions of portraiture and representationalism that seem to have been so central to the legal, medical, and institutional photography that Tagg describes.

What is the historical basis for the scientific cinema's nonpictorial mode of representation? Frank suggests that Marey's techniques of motion recording and analysis, which came to be known as "the graphic method," had the stature of "a new language," the bearing of which is expressed in Borell's assertion that

> as the graphic method evolved, a new conception of the body emerged. Analysis of separate physiological events, the reductionist approach, revealed the interrelatedness of these events and the body's complex control mechanisms. By the second quarter of the twentieth century, in fact, these homeostatic mechanisms

had become a major focus for biological research. Moreover, pharmacological studies had also matured: experimental analysis of the effect of drugs on physiological processes illuminated the nature of those processes, as well as suggested more precise biological tests for individual drugs.[34]

This "language" of physiology incorporated Marey's technique of chrono-photography and was the basis of Auguste Lumière's laboratory work in pharmacology and medical biology after 1901. From the perspective of film studies, the identification of physiology's methodology as a "graphic language" has a certain resonance. It evokes the broad application of semiotics in the study of the cinema.[35] However, the studies of Borell and others have tended to focus on the work process of physiologists and their methods and instruments rather than on texts (the images, graphs, charts, and analyses produced through the method) and their reception and use. Throughout this volume, I trace a history of the medical and scientific motion study that draws from both of these disciplines (film studies and the history of medicine and science). In order to underscore the place of the popular in this conjuncture, I conclude this chapter by returning to my claim that the film motion study is more than simply a technique of nineteenth-century science and medicine or a subgenre of the documentary tradition. As I demonstrate in this chapter's concluding discussion of the early cinema genre of the facial-expression film, the fascination with physiological and technological spectacles of "life" was a transversal phenomenon, cutting across popular, public, and professional visual cultures.

Tom Gunning has made a case for a genre of the early cinema, which he calls a "cinema of attractions," that provides some useful ways of thinking about how the graphic method intersected with a physiological tradition of popular cinema. Gunning discusses the facial-expression film, a category that includes the Edison/Dickson 1894 *Kinetoscopic Record of a Sneeze*, as an example of this cinema of attraction. He suggests this mode is evident in pre-1906 films characterized in part by use of the close-up, the actor's look at the camera, and absence of narrative—a style centered on the performer's act of displaying bodily movement. "A more primal fascination with the act of display" is the suggested cultural motivation for the reception of this type of film.[36]

Perhaps nowhere is the popular cinema's debt to experimental physiology and its surveillant gaze more clear than in the *Kinetoscopic Record of a Sneeze*. The film documents the moment of the physiological act of the sneeze, an event that induces the momentary cessation of the heartbeat. The sneeze perfectly suits physiology's interest in documenting the changes that occur in a physiological process. Further, it represents an instance of involuntary movement, an activity beyond the control of the observer. As Linda Williams notes (citing Gordon Hendricks), the film was made at the request of a reporter for *Harper's Weekly*, a request that specified, in Williams' words, "a pretty young woman who would have lent prurient interest to the involuntary comic act of a sneeze."[37] The film, which ultimately featured not a "pretty woman" but Edison's laboratory assistant Fred Ott, was featured in *Harper's* in a series of frame enlargements. These images evoke no convention more than the film motion study reproduced for frame analysis in science and medical journals of the period (see figure 1.1).

Gunning suggests that viewers experienced a physical response to this type of image, a visceral and immediate reaction that carried a certain immediacy and charge not elicited by, for example, films composed of long shots and less invested in the display of bodily events. He contrasts the "primitive" spectatorial immediacy afforded by this kind of film with the hypothetically more distanced and analytical spectatorial position associated with the later narrative cinema. But here Gunning seems to confuse the immediacy of the act portrayed—the image of uncontrolled motor activity in the film body—with the production of perceptual immediacy "in" the viewer. He assumes an identificatory link between images of physiological acts (sneezing, exercising, grimacing) and the spectator.

In the case of films such as the American Mutoscope and Biograph Company's *Female Facial Expressions* (1902) and *Photographing a Female Crook* (1904; figure 1.2), or Edison's *Electrocuting an Elephant* (1903), we also find physiological events presented in close-up as spectacles of corporeality. However, it can be argued that such close-ups and foregrounded bodily movement likely would have repelled their audiences.[38] In *Female Facial Expressions* and *Photographing a Female Crook*, for example, we see female bodies resisting conformity to "normal" physiology. In the former, a woman is shot in close-up as she contorts her face for the camera. In the latter, a woman "crook" is restrained by male officers before the camera as she grimaces, distorting her features (presumably in order to render her photo ID unrecognizable). Whereas in the former film the grimacing of the woman demonstrates a resistance to standards of female beauty, the "female crook" demonstrates the resistance of filmed subjects to the visual classification of their bodies as a mode of social control. One might say that this type of film might more accurately be dubbed a cinema of repulsion. Ironically, these popular expression films represent attempts to undercut the association between expression and meaning. The films both amuse and repel precisely because they represent subjects attempting to escape normative bodily conventions (for example, visual beauty and recognizability). In some ways, the spectator whose pleasure in the image hinges on an enjoyment of the spectacle of this refusal of representation, or on the thrill of repulsion (in the case of Edison's *Electrocuting an Elephant*, for example), is not unlike the spectator of the scientific film motion study, the scientist who takes pleasure in observing often aberrant and repulsive physiological processes. The films of Gunning's

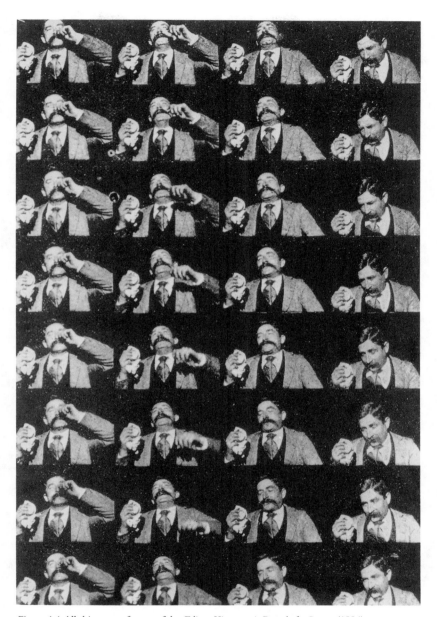

Figure 1.1 All thirty-two frames of the *Edison Kinetoscopic Record of a Sneeze* (1894).

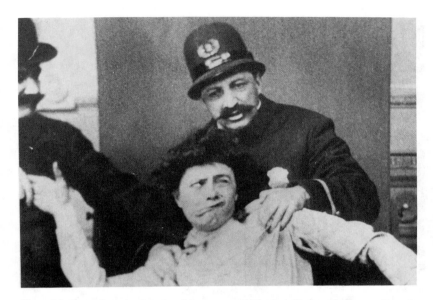

Figure 1.2. Frame from the American Mutoscope and Biograph Company's *Photographing a Female Crook* (1904).

cinema of attractions ultimately seem to demand a spectator for whom disavowal undercuts the immediacy of the sight of a body that refuses self-regulation. The mode of the physiological motion study thus seems to appear, incongruously enough, in the popular cinema, where it invites the spectator to participate in the "scientific" fascination with the execution of "life."

CHAPTER 2

"Experiments of Destruction": Cinematic Inscriptions of Physiology

THE FRENCH PHYSIOLOGIST CLAUDE BERNARD stated in 1878 that "there is an arrangement in the living being, a kind of regulated activity, which must never be neglected, because it is in truth the most striking characteristic of living beings."[1] Though Bernard never used photographic motion studies in his experiments, serial photography (and, later, cinematography) clearly suggested to other physiologists of his generation the potential not only for observing but for intervening in the dynamic "regulated activity" that, for physiologists, best characterized the living beings they studied.

The ideological implications of observation of and intervention in the physiological "arrangement" of the "living being" are demonstrated strikingly by the 1903 Edison Manufacturing Company film *Electrocuting an Elephant*. This film and the events surrounding its production reveal the degree to which physiology and its drive to regulate life and death had become a part of public culture by the turn of the century. A popular attraction at Coney Island's Luna Park was Topsy, a four-ton elephant captured in Africa and brought to the United States, where she lived in captivity for twenty-eight years. Topsy's popularity increased dramatically when she killed three men, to the horror and amazement of Luna Park spectators. An uncontrollable, man-killing beast was a much more exciting attraction than a docile animal. The Luna Park authorities decided, however, that Topsy posed too much of a risk alive. The execution that they plotted proved to be an attraction almost more popular, and undoubtedly more dramatic, than the display of the living animal had been. Luna Park officials commissioned the Edison Manufacturing Company to build an apparatus for the electrocution of the elephant. This was no simple task, given the weight and perceived danger of the elephant. A station designed to house equipment for administering a six-thousand-volt shock was constructed a hundred feet away from the designated execution site. Electrical wires linked the structure to electrodes implanted in a set of wooden sandals designed to fit Topsy's large feet. The site, which amply accommodated spectators, was outfitted with an Edison movie-camera rig. A *New York World* reporter described the scene:

> While fifteen hundred persons looked on in breathless excitement, an electric bolt of 6,000 volts sent Topsy, the man-killing elephant, staggering to the ground yesterday at Luna Park, Coney Island. With her own life [she] paid for the lives of the three men she had killed.
>
> It was all over in a moment. . . . The current was turned on . . . and quick as a flash the colossal form of the elephant stiffened forward, then quivered in the throes of the mighty bolt, sinking finally to the ground without a groan. (Figure 2.1)

I begin this chapter on physiological experimentation and the cinema with an anecdote about a production of a popular motion picture company, a film that documents a public spectacle of punishment by death, in order to demonstrate that physiology, the science of living processes and functions, was not limited to the intrainstitutional practice of the scientific laboratory. Through events and films like the one described, the regulated physiological activity that Bernard insisted must never be neglected by physiologists became the object of rapt public attention. The Edison Manufacturing Company must have banked on the fact that in 1903 audiences would have paid not only to observe an intervention in the "regulated activity" of the "living being" but to study this intervention again and again on film, just as the laboratory scientist might watch just such a film over and over to analyze the execution of "life." The one-minute *Electrocuting an Elephant* documents the moment of the elephant's death. But, more importantly, it also documents public fascination with scientific technology and its capacity to determine the course of life and death in living beings, even those as physically and symbolically powerful as the elephant. The film, and the documentation surrounding its production, is evidence of a widespread popular interest in the power of technology to regulate and discipline bodies. Further, it demonstrates that the motion picture functioned as a means for lay-audience participation in the "scientific" pleasure of conducting visual analysis and thereby vicariously exerting control over a living being's life and death. Indeed, it is worth noting that the object of this public "experiment" was a specimen of colonial plunder inserted within a spectacle designed to entertain fantasies of colonial authority. At Luna Park, the elephants were also used in stagings of "exotic" cultures. In turning from a docile and compliant animal into a violent beast, Topsy became the object of displaced Western anxieties about resistance to colonial authority.[2]

This chapter introduces some of the methods and techniques of physiological viewing as a disciplinary and regulatory power, techniques that are considered in closer detail in subsequent chapters. In the following pages I proceed through descriptions of a series of moments in the history of scien-

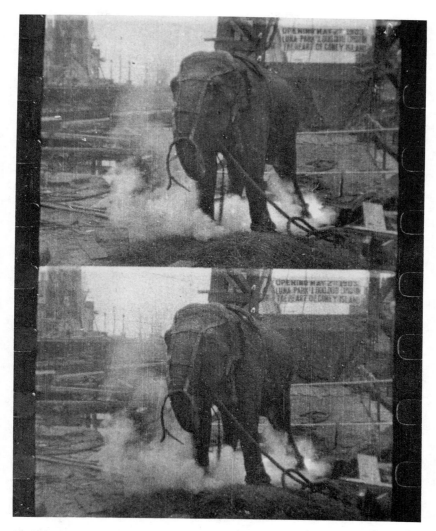

Figure 2.1. Frames from *Electrocuting an Elephant,* Edison Manufacturing Company, 1903. Photograph by Patrick G. Loughney, courtesy American Federation of the Arts.

tific visual and quantitative analysis. I begin by noting two examples of early medical film motion studies to demonstrate how the fascination with movement and interior, invisible processes in the early scientific cinema was bound up with the logic of the kymograph and its graphic, linear trace—a kind of "seeing" that differs in important ways from other modes of cinematic and pictorial spectatorship. I then turn to the work of Bernard to consider the relationship of technology and body in the science of physiology. Clearly some physiologists regarded optical recording devices as a means particularly well suited to the task of charting and measuring movement. But Bernard's methodology suggests that the experimental apparatus, a setup in which many other physiologists would later include the motion-picture camera, was understood not only to document but to alter the "arrangement" of the living process under study. In other words, as a laboratory technique, cinematography did not simply record or document movement; as we shall see in later chapters, it regulated, disciplined, and transformed the body studied. Finally, this chapter considers some of the work of Marey's students and followers, physiologists who regarded cinematography as a technology uniquely suited to the laboratory culture of physiology and its graphic encoding of living processes. In the experiments described in this last section, we see the degree to which the "arrangement" of the living being studied is regulated and disciplined by the experimental apparatus. I conclude this chapter by returning briefly to the case of Topsy and the Edison film of her electrocution in order to emphasize the crucial similarities between certain public media spectacles of life and death and the cinematic study of living beings in laboratory experimentation.[3]

Charting Interior Physiology: The Film Motion Study in the Late Nineteenth Century

Many nineteenth-century American and European scientists regarded the cinematic devices introduced by the Lumières, Edison, and others in 1895 not as new inventions but as improved versions of the photographic apparatuses of Marey and Muybridge. Cinematography was quickly incorporated into laboratory practice as an experimental technique, to be used alongside a range of techniques of inscription and visualization (including kymography, microscopy, and photography). For example, in 1897 the Scottish physician John Macintyre took a rapid succession of X-ray photographs of the movements of a frog's leg, rephotographed this series onto a strip of motion picture film, and loop-projected this film on a cinematograph (figure 2.2). And in 1898, the Viennese researcher Ludwig Braun surgically exposed a living dog's heart and filmed its contractions (figure 2.3).[4] Early film motion studies

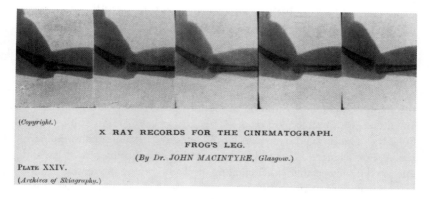

Figure 2.2. Frames from John Macintyre's X-ray cinematography of a frog's leg in motion. Reproduced in *Archives of Clinical Skiagraphy* 1, no. 4 (1897).

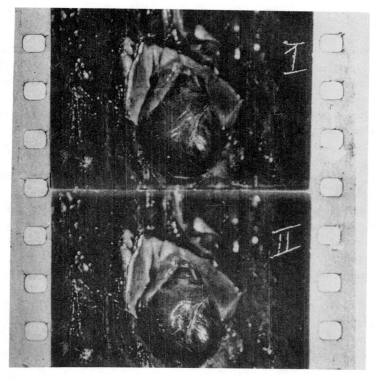

Figure 2.3. Frames from Ludwig Braun's cinematography of a dog's beating heart, as they appear in Braun, *Über Herzbewegung und Herzstoss* (Jena, 1898).

such as these demonstrate that Marey's mistrust of cinematography as a physiological technique (discussed later in this chapter) was not at all universal.

Macintyre describes his film in terms of a standard scientific agenda. He was, in his words, "obtaining rapid exposures with a view to recording the movements of organs within the body" (in order eventually to use this process for medical diagnosis in humans, for example).[5] In contradiction to this expressed practical aim, one of the film's first public screenings was for an audience assembled on Ladies' Night at the Glasgow Philosophical Society—a group whose interests would not have been limited to the purely medical or scientific. Films like Macintyre's drew the interest of lay audiences, who viewed them as fascinating displays of living movement. But the images that were so entertaining were often neither pictorial nor narrative in form. Lacking plot, characters, and conventional representational form, Macintyre's film was simply a close-up sequence of the movements of a single joint of a frog's leg. Judging from the film frames Macintyre published in a journal essay, the moving radiographic image must have appeared to its audience as a flat, schematic, and linear silhouette. The image received with such interest by the Ladies' Night audience was something closer to a kymographic trace than to a photograph; apparently, the graphic images of nineteenth-century physiology easily crossed over to the genre of popular visual spectacle.

The flat, schematic quality of radiological imaging makes Macintyre's film a convenient illustration of the tendency to the flat and graphic that would dominate in the physiological cinema. Braun's film of a dog's exposed beating heart, however, does not lend itself as readily to this analysis because it conforms more closely to conventional photographic properties. Unlike the X-ray image, which is recorded without a photographic lens, Braun's image was rendered through a standard photographic lens. However, the use to which Braun put his images suggests that he, like Macintyre, regarded his film as something akin to a kymographic trace, a graphic register of change over time.

Braun, like Macintyre, viewed his filmstrip as a series of flat, static images, as if composed on a page (as they are displayed, in fact, in his book). He measured and analyzed differences occurring between each pair of frames, such as changes in shape and displacements of shadow marking the heart's contractions. These measurements provided him with new quantitative data through which to analyze the physiological characteristics of the heartbeat. Apparently, what interested Braun was not primarily the spectacle of the heart in motion but the capacity of the moving image to be stopped, measured, and quantified. If he "saw" the heart's movement in the cinema image, he saw it in terms of static, graphic, and measurable indices. Like Edison's *Electrocuting an Elephant*, Braun's film is a precise, incremental index of life and death—a register that is, in very important ways, a graphic trace and not a moving picture.

The films of Macintyre and Braun suggest that the physiological cinema is marked by a drive not only to segment, to measure, and to quantify movement, but also to render visible parts of the living body that were previously considered to be too interiorized, too minute, or too private to be seen by the researcher's unaided eye. The imaging of the body's interior space in medicine and science has suggested to some scholars a narrative of Western advancement characterized by technology's prosthetic augmentation of the sensory powers already built in, as it were, to the scientific observer's body.[6] This argument suggests that devices designed to visualize physiological processes in effect enhanced researchers' perceptual powers, extending the observer's epistemological domain into previously uncharted territories—an Enlightenment project that continues in today's medical imaging technologies.

However, Braun's use of cinema film—a kind of use typical of physiological cinema at the turn of the century and after—suggests that the augmentation of sight, and imaging as such, may not have been the central agendas in modernist science's optical invasion of the body's interior space. Rather than simply augmenting the senses of the scientific observer, cinematography supplemented or replaced sensory perception. The inscriptions of data produced through techniques like kymography or cinematography in the physiological laboratory replaced the sensory observations of the physician or technician as a privileged source of scientific knowledge. Jonathan Crary argues this case with regard to physiological optics in the early decades of the nineteenth century. He states of contemporary visual practices:

> Most of the historically important functions of the human eye are being supplanted by practices in which visual images no longer have any reference to an observer in a "real," optically perceived world. If these images can be said to refer to anything, it is to millions of bits of electronic mathematical data. Increasingly, visuality will be situated on a cybernetic and electromagnetic terrain where abstract visual and linguistic elements coincide and are consumed, circulated and exchanged globally.[7]

The subsuming and dispersing of sight in the postcolonial global knowledge systems Crary alludes to occurs not in spite of, but precisely through, the popularization of newer visual technologies like ultrasound, MRI, and PET scanning.[8] These technologies, and their paradoxically antivisual tendency, can be traced back to Marey's apparatuses for optically measuring and analyzing the body, and to the cephalometers, calipers, and craniometers used by mid- to late-nineteenth century scientists to inscribe racial and sexual difference in quantitative terms.[9] As Borell has pointed out, Marey's techniques (and, I would add, Braun's and Macintyre's) precede the numerous more recent imaging modalities used in contemporary laboratories and hospitals to track human physiology—noninvasive diagnostic imaging techniques such as echocardiography, video monitoring of bioelectric impulses, fiberoptic motion imaging of endoscopic investigations of the uterine walls or the gall bladder, or the optical tracking of radioactive tracer molecules introduced into the bloodstream.

In order to understand the cultural implications of this "antivisual" and graphic tendency in medical imaging that can be traced from Macintyre and Braun to the present, it is necessary to look back on some of the nonvisual techniques used by Marey to track bodily movement. Marey's early recording devices are noted for their connection to later noninvasive modes of physiological analysis. François Dagognet, in his book-length study of Marey, quotes from an essay by Marey that considers explicitly the invasive method of vivisection:

> Vivisection in itself is inadequate for the study of biology; all it does is lay bare the phenomenon . . . . All it reveals to our senses is what they can directly perceive. But you have seen in physics how little our senses tell us, so that we are constantly obliged to use apparatuses in order to analyze things.[10]

Even when Marey "invaded" the interior of the body, his purpose was not simply to open it up for observation. Consider, for example, the following example of an early experiment of Marey's. Decades before Braun's cinema film of a dog's beating heart, Marey and J. B. A. Chauveau inserted air-filled ampules into the chambers of a horse's beating heart. These ampules were connected by tubes to a kymograph, which registered a cardiographic trace of pressure changes in each chamber. This linear record of the relative movements of each chamber was inscribed by a stylus onto a roll of graphite-coated paper mounted onto a slowly rotating cylinder (figure 2.4).[11] By tapping directly into the heart, Marey and Chauveau were able to measure and quantify with great precision the movements characteristic of a living heart. The magnitude of this experiment is clear when one recalls that autopsy was the chief investigatory technique of the nineteenth century. With a living body taking the place of the corpse in their laboratory investigation of the body's interior, Marey and Chauveau were able to supplement information about cardiac anatomy with detailed physiological information—data regarding function, process, and movement of the heart during life. This experiment marks a dual shift in methodology: a shift toward movement as a characteristic state of the body, and a shift toward graphic inscription as a means of recording interior processes. Significantly, these shifts simultaneously mark a move toward implanting a technology of observation directly into the body studied—a technique that joins technology and the living body rather than using technology to sacrifice the body for the sake of analysis. Marey and Chauveau had devised an apparatus in which the technology and

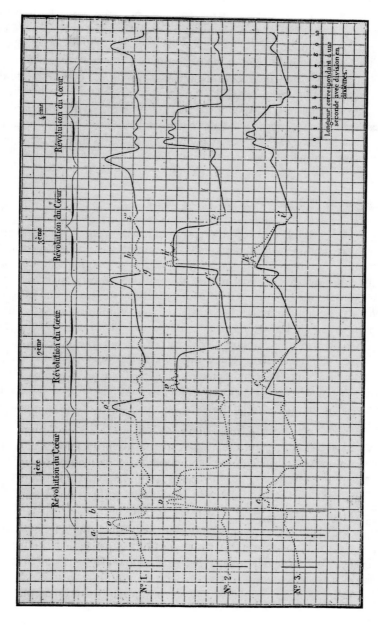

Figure 2.4. Comparative tracing of cardiographic pressure changes recorded by J. B. A. Chauveau and Etienne-Jules Marey. From Marey, *La Méthode graphique* (Paris, 1878)

the life form it interrogated were made into a generative and interdependent system. As the horse's body motored the inscription device, so the kymographic inscription reconfigured the conception of the living body from within, rendering it an ordered living system—a system best represented by graphical, temporal forms like the calibrated kymographic line or the incremental cinematic image, for example. Physiology's laboratory instruments and human physiology thus became mutually constitutive processes. But before demonstrating the place of film motion study in this relation, I will expand briefly on a text by Claude Bernard in order to clarify the place of observation in this context, and the crucial differences between Bernard's deadly methodology of vivisection and Marey's emphasis on generating living processes through technologies of inscription.

Bernard's "Experiments of Destruction"

Bernard, a physiologist who was well known to both Auguste Lumière and Marey, gave considerable attention in his writings to the issue of experimental method. Although he did not use photography or film himself, his work is a useful source for considering the place of optical instruments like the movie camera in physiology. His 1865 *Introduction to the Study of Experimental Medicine* sets out a distinction between the mode of observation and that of experimentation in laboratory practice. Bernard opposes the term "observation," which consists in "noting everything normal and regular," to the term "experiment," which acknowledges the "variation or disturbance that an investigator brings into the conditions of natural phenomena." I quote the following example of what Bernard calls "experiments of destruction" to provide some sense of what he means by the investigator's causing "variation or disturbance" in the internal functioning of a phenomenon:

> We suppress an organ in the living subject, by a section or ablation; and from the disturbance produced in the whole organism or in a special function, we deduce the function of the missing organism. This essentially analytic, experimental method is put into practice every day in physiology. For instance, anatomy has taught us that two principal nerves diverge in the face: the facial (seventh cranial) and the trigeminal (fifth cranial); to learn their functions, they were cut, one at a time. The result showed that section of the facial nerve brings about loss of movement, and section of the trigeminal, loss of sensation, from which it was concluded that the facial is the motor nerve of the face, and the trigeminal the sensory nerve.[12]

In this instance, it is only through the stopping of a "normal" activity—its suppression or destruction—that the function of an activity can be known. This foregrounding of a phenomenon's absence in the study of its function has important implications for sensory perception, and especially for the sense of sight. Bernard claims that his method makes natural phenomena "present themselves in circumstances or conditions in which nature does not show them."[13] However, in the experiment described above, Bernard's intervention—the severing of a nerve—precludes the potential for nerve activity to "present itself." What is ultimately shown is nothing more than an absence, a body stripped of its capacity to perform the function in question. The phenomenon emerges as an imperceptible differential between a past event and its absence. "Life," then, is something perceptible only through a kind of rigor mortis.

Merriley Borell discusses instruments used in the nineteenth and twentieth centuries for the analysis of physiological processes as part of a project of "extending the senses" of the medical and scientific observer.[14] As the example of Marey and Chauveau's kymographic tracing of a horse's heartbeat shows, the kymograph registered precise graphic, quantitative data of the body's interior, minute, and transient oscillations and responses. But is the instrument's mediation necessarily an extension of the physiologist's senses, as Borell suggests? Bernard's description suggests not. For Bernard, experimental observation transgressed the boundaries between observation of a phenomenon and the very life of the phenomenon. The severing of a nerve is without question an intervention in the course of nerve action. Borell notes that "Ludwig's kymographion and Helmholz's myograph both involved invasive surgical procedures: the kymographion requiring direct connection with a blood vessel by a catheter, the myograph recording from an isolated muscle."[15] To what degree did such early observational procedures facilitate Bernard's stated agenda of aiding the "self-presentation of a system in nature," when the act of observation intervenes in the course of living systems? The kymograph can be said to highlight the limits of the observer's sensory powers insofar as it corrects and disciplines empirical observation by providing more detailed data about internal functions. What is extended, perhaps, is not the observer's senses but the living process of the body studied, and the epistemological domain of the apparatus in the generation of "life." In the case of Marey and Chauveau's experiment described above, the phenomenon that is ostensibly observed fails to function within the limits of a given sensory register (such as sight). What is "observed" is not the phenomenon but an encoded inscription of an activity functioning beyond sensory thresholds, or an activity whose life can be measured only against its physiological condition of death. Far from prosthetically extending the senses, the kymograph and its linear, digitally encoded image fills the vacuum in signification produced by the failure of sensory observation.

Although late-nineteenth-century physiology is noted for the use of all forms of mechanical and optical instrumentation, and Bernard is known to have made use of such equipment, he mentions only visual and tactile observation. His experiment on the nerves is a relatively simple one, its data relatively straightforward, demonstrating that a social technology does not require complex hardware. The failure of the senses need not entail the extension or replacement of the faculties of sight, touch, or smell with machines. Bernard's experiment illustrates quite clearly the idea behind the incorporation of technology within living systems, even when that "technology" is the experimenter's eye or the test subject's nervous system. Bernard implicates observation in an act that quite radically breaks from the use of seeing to simply measure, or to know, a phenomenon. In the following passage he discusses the sense of touch not simply in terms of its potential for observation but in terms of its potential to alter its object physically:

> This definition of experiment necessarily assumes that experimenters must be able to touch the body on which they wish to act, whether by destroying it or by altering it, so as to learn the part which it plays in the phenomena of nature. . . . It is on this very possibility of acting, or not acting, on a body that the distinction will exclusively rest between sciences called sciences of observation and sciences called experimental.[16]

This privileging of the sense of touch—the assertion that "experimenters must be able to touch the body on which they wish to act"—initially seems to advance direct observation as a mode of investigation or measurement. Among the senses, touch would seem to remain most bound to the empirical immediacy, for instance. Palpation, diagnosis by means of touch, is not usually understood to implement a change in the body or object under study. However, Bernard considers touch capable of moving beyond noninvasive observation. Touching is no longer a neutral intermediary between physician/experimenter and body/object; touch constitutes "action on the body" insofar as it alters the object it investigates. Touching, looking, and other sensory acts performed to observe phenomena are now recognized as agents acting not only on the body but in and through it, as instruments implicated in the course of the life process studied.

For Bernard, this shift in the action of the senses is historical and progressive, not biological. He does not imply that the senses themselves have altered materially, but that their instrumental uses are evolving historically. The progress of Western scientific medicine, then, is bound up in the compounding of the physiological act of observation, experimental instruments, and the physiological systems studied in a complex technological apparatus through which "experiments of destruction" are conducted. One can no longer speak of bodies or objects of knowledge without acknowledging the in-built technologies through which their health and life are regulated and disciplined.

How was the Cinématographe incorporated in this experimental apparatus; how did it intervene in the life of the bodies it was used to study? In the remainder of this chapter I attempt to elaborate a kind of prehistory and early history of the physiological film motion study by weaving together a series of moments that can be regarded as formative in the development of a disciplinary scientific visual apparatus. Thus far I have suggested that in turn-of-the-century science the serial photograph and the cinematic film functioned as parts of a system of representation whose precedents were most significantly nonvisual instruments of measurement and quantification, and that this history suggests that the cinema has been informed in crucial ways by scientific modes of seeing and knowing. In the pages that follow, I consider the use of photography in nineteenth-century astronomy and the use of cinematography in early twentieth-century physiology as moments in a history of the cinema as a technique for disciplining populations and bodies—a technique grounded in an ideological insistence on science's ability not to destroy but to enliven its bodies and subjects through technological means. The examples presented below are intended to introduce and historicize this book's broader case for a physiological cinema whose optical mode of knowledge consists in a transformation of observation and the documentary mode of representation toward experimentation and the physical transformation of the individual and social body.

Photography as Graphic System

Thus far I have hinted at the role of graphic inscription in a disciplinary mode of representation. But what is the specific relationship between graphic inscription and the cultural agenda of disciplining and regulating bodies? What are the cultural mechanisms through which inscription becomes a disciplinary force, and on and among whom is this force exerted? Early uses of the photographic camera as an instrument of measurement and quantification provide a useful example through which to begin to address these questions.

Outlining the merits of the daguerreotype in a report to the French Chamber of Deputies in 1839, Dominique François Arago, the head of a major Parisian astronomical observatory, stressed the scientific uses of this new technology. He began by describing the difficulties laboratory scientists were experiencing in their attempts to conduct time-based comparisons:

> An important branch of the science of observation and calculation, that which deals with the intensity of light, photometry, has so far made little progress. The physicist has no difficulty in determining the comparative intensities of two lights, one next to the other and both simultaneously visible; but there are only imperfect means for making such a comparison when the condition of simultaneity is lacking, as when a light which is now visible is to be compared with another light, which will not be visible until after the first light has disappeared.[17]

Having presented the representation of temporality as a procedural snag, Arago went on to propose the daguerreotype as a solution. He suggested that a series of photographs be taken from a fixed position with the appearance of each light, and that these images be used to measure time and distance. Clearly, the type of image Arago described is markedly different from the pictorial landscape, portrait, or still life associated with the daguerreotype. In his account, the light record is presented as a graphic and digital index, an image that forgoes the conventions of perspective built into the photographic lens. Prefiguring the temporal unit of the cinema frame, the light-intensity indices function together as a quantitative register of temporal difference, much like a series of film frames.

Arago's hypothetical setup bears an unmistakable likeness to the scene people might have witnessed in astronomical observatories during this same period. He described the appearance of points of light at temporal intervals, an image suggesting the appearance and disappearance of stars in the sky. This particular setting—a lateral field in which factors like depth of field and surface detail are rendered null by the extreme degree of distance between star and observer—is a scene that fails to lend itself to such painterly and photographic conventions as perspective, foreshortening, and modeling. Indeed, Arago explicitly stated that the daguerreotype might be used to make photographic maps of the stars. "In a few moments of time," he speculated, "one can achieve the longest and most difficult project in astronomy."[18]

The use of the daguerreotype as graphic register that Arago proposed recalls Carl Ludwig's kymograph, with its graphical and digital record of change. Indeed, Borell describes the very earliest electrocardiographs as instruments involving the recording of an optical signal onto a photographic plate to create a graphic index much like the image Arago described.[19] Almost forty years after Arago's report on the daguerreotype, the Norwegian astronomer Pierre J. C. Janssen produced a photographic apparatus for astronomical measurement. Janssen placed a barrellike camera holding a circular, sensitized metal photographic plate in the focal plane of a telescope. A clock mechanism rotated the plate by small increments at equal intervals, exposing successive images along the plate's periphery. Each plate held forty-eight separate images, each exposed for seventy-two seconds. Janssen analyzed this register of temporal change to gauge the velocity of planetary motion.

This astronomical revolver is widely regarded as a precursor to Marey's chronophotographic gun. But here we see that it is also directly indebted to a tradition of scientific motion recording that can be traced back to the origins of photography. Although the measurement of the circulation of the blood or the movement of human and animal bodies may seem a far cry from the measurement of the movement of astral bodies, the two methods have more in common than would appear. In both operations, a "moving body" is tracked. And, more importantly, the body of the observer is disciplined and regulated within the mechanism of the overall apparatus. This point is demonstrated by Simon Shaffer in his analysis of the role of the human observer in Charles Wheatstone's astronomical chronoscope (constructed in 1840) and the chronographs used by Greenwich and Harvard astronomers in the 1850s. Shaffer describes the Greenwich chronoscopes, instruments for graphically charting the movements of the stars, as instruments that

> involved the combination of the motion of an "artificial star" whose speed of transit could be standardized, with a recording device in which the initiation of a galvanic signal could record the elapsed time as measured by astronomers under test. [The British astronomer G. B.] Airy's recording device included a uniformly rotating drum and a powerful electromagnet to produce a calibrated trace; the "artificial star" was typically produced as a point image of a bright light.[20]

Bernard expressed the view that astronomy could not progress into its experimental stage because it was so tightly bound to distanced observation. The telescope augmented what could be perceived by the eye but, he explained, could not control the course of the distant astral movement it rendered visible.[21] Though action on the "bodies" of the stars was an impossibility, managers of astronomical observatories were nevertheless successfully acting on the bodies of their human observers, minimizing the subjective factor of their embodied sensory observations. The locus of experimentation had shifted from the distant astral body to the body of the observer. Shaffer describes a scene in which human computers standing watch in observatories closely traced the movements of stars and recorded their observations. These recordings were then analyzed by the managers of these astronomical sites— men who did not actually observe the stars themselves. These managers subjected the human computers' performance to rigorous surveillance, checking their figures against proven norms and data derived from the chronoscope. Shaffer states that the complex electromagnetic technology of Airy's apparatus "intervened between observer and image," its artificial stars and galvanic clocks calibrating "the disciplined performance of the observer." But the observers' performance was also calibrated by their superiors. In Shaffer's words, astronomical computers were "inspected by their superiors with as much concern as were the stars themselves."[22]

In the astronomical observatory Shaffer describes, instrumental and managerial intervention constituted a kind of action or experimentation on the embodied vision of the observer. Incorporated in the measurement instrument, the observer's own physiological faculties were managed and regulated through a reflexive and internal control system. Observation became a function performed through a complex technological apparatus.[23] Like the Panopticon that Foucault describes, the observatory offered the potential for a reflexive supervision of its own mechanisms. "An inspector arriving unexpectedly at the centre of the Panopticon," Foucault explains, "will be able to judge at a glance, without anything being concealed from him, how the entire establishment is functioning."[24] However, there is a crucial difference in the operation of the two systems as Shaffer and Foucault describe them. The Panopticon operates most centrally through visuality. It is a system of surveillance in which, Foucault tells us, the director controls its operation by spying "on all the employees he has under his supervision." Indeed, from the central tower, one might even "observe the director himself."[25] But the inspection of the astronomical observer takes place through very different management techniques, methods that do not give visuality such a pivotal place in the disciplinary apparatus. Shaffer states that the inspection of the observers took place in large part through a comparative study of human and technological data, the performance of artificial stars and galvanic clocks calibrating the performance of the observer. Thus it is in the process of analyzing and comparing data on human and technological performance that disciplinary action takes place, not in the act of observation itself.

The foregrounding of data inscription, analysis, and instrumental regulation over the act of observation has critical implications for my historicization of the daguerreotype. In astronomy, the observing human computer functioned, in effect, as a component of the recording instrument. Much like the chronoscope, the human computers were meant to inscribe. Computers and chronoscopes recorded data numerically and graphically. As Arago seems to suggest in his report to the Chamber of Deputies, the making of graphic indices was as legitimate a project of photography as the production of pictorial scenes. Indeed, Arago implies that the photosensitive plate is, in fact, a record of the forces that expose it. He claims that, if exposure patterns on a plate confirm variations in the intensity of the source of exposure throughout the day,

> the meteorologist will have a new element to record in his tables, and to the ancient observations as to the state of the thermometer, barometer, and hygrometer and the visibility of the air they [meteorologists] will have to add another element, which these early instruments do not indicate. It will be necessary to take into consideration an absorption of a peculiar character which cannot be without influence on many other phenomena, perhaps even on those belonging to the fields of physiology and medicine.[26]

Underlying Arago's statement is the assumption that the photosensitive plate, like the kymograph or the thermometer, is uniquely suited to the recording and quantitative analysis of movements and forces—an agenda that in no way mandated the use of the photograph as a pictorial register of static scenes but suggested its use as a graphic record of time and movement.[27] Nowhere is this potential for photography as a graphic method more thoroughly demonstrated than in the chronophotography of Marey. In the following section, I take a closer look at the function of graphic inscription in the time and motion studies of Marey.

Chronophotography and the Rejection of the Lens

For Marey, the logic of embodied sight incorporated in his chronophotographic apparatus presented some serious methodological obstacles. Most significantly, the optical geometry of the camera's lens was in conflict with the kymograph's quantitative logic. As Comolli has argued, it was precisely the elements of perspective and foreshortening introduced into chronophotography by the photographic lens and plate that complicated Marey's graphic method.[28] Marey went to great lengths to reduce the distortions in measurement brought about by the imposition of lenticular perspective and tonal gradation. His celebrated graphical studies of locomotion will serve as my case in point.

Many of Marey's photographic studies at the Physiological Station in Paris were shot against what appears in the photographs to be a flat black backdrop. However, F. A. Talbot, author of an early history of the cinema, points out that what appeared to be a flat wall was in fact a deep cavity (not unlike Edison's Black Maria). "The cavity may be likened to a shed," Talbot explains, "the front wall of which is removed and the whole interior blackened" with velvet, pitch, and a flat black paint.[29] Paradoxically, this deep space was essential to the rendering of an apparently flat backdrop, eliminating the light reflection that an actual flat surface would produce.

In one study of human locomotion done at this site, Marey clothed a human body in black from head to foot. This costume was marked with graphic white lines and points, creating a kind of skeletal framework on the exterior of the subject's body. Filmed walking against the backdrop of the dark shed, the black-clothed body in effect disappeared from the image field—that is, except for the schematic skeletal lines that marked its limbs and torso. The fixed-plate sequence produced in the study of the man in black appears as an abstract series of linear registers—a skeletal image that functions, in much the same way as does the kymographic line or Macintyre's radiographic film of a frog's joint, as a graphic map of relational points across a virtually two-dimensional space (figures 2.5 and 2.6). Further demonstrating the penchant for flatness that is so evident in this series is the fact that Marey further compensated for the "problem" of computing dimensional lenticular space by devising mathematical equations to "correct" spatial irregularities in the image due to the curvature of the lens and resultant variations in lens-to-object distance across the image field.

In his study of cinema and technology, Steve Neale also presents the man-

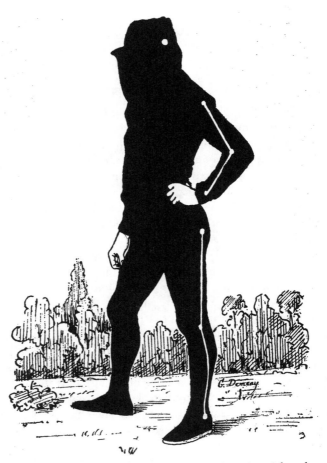

in-black series as evidence of Marey's opposition to the pictorial codes of photographic representation:

> Marey was even more insistent [than his U.S. counterpart Eadweard Muybridge] that research and analysis entailed not only breaking with age-old conventions of representation and perception, but also breaking with the perceptions of photography itself, the very ideology in which it was caught and which it hitherto had been used to support. He pushed it even further beyond the threshold of appearance by deconstructing its surface verisimilitude, its ability to produce a dense, detailed, homogeneous image. In order to trace the shapes and patterns of movement, he did everything possible to break down the sensuous density of the photograph, posing his subjects in black against a carefully constructed black surface, with only white abstract shapes on various portions of the limbs to mark stages of movement, replacing the seamless analog of the conventional photographic image with posed, constructed and specifically arbitrary signs.[30]

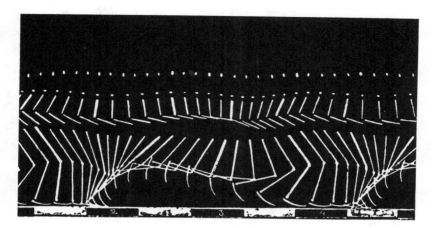

Figure 2.6. Diagram taken from a photographic study of human gait. From Etienne-Jules Marey, *Le mouvement* (Paris, 1894).

Clearly Marey went to great lengths to eliminate from many of his images the pictorial and spatial elements associated with the photographic lens. But what are the cultural implications of this proclivity for flatness and graphic inscription? I would argue that his signs were no more arbitrary than the analogic photograph—that his mode of graphic inscription functioned within the terms of the graphic method, as a particular kind of ideological technique.

A comparison of the study of the man-in-black series with other examples of late-nineteenth-century anatomical and physiological visual analysis helps to demonstrate the similarities and differences among the analogic photographic system from which Marey distanced himself and the chronophotographic method he embraced. Sekula has described the conjuncture of photography and phrenology in 1896, in Mathew Brady's work on "criminal jurisprudence," and in the slightly later photographic studies of criminals by Alphonse Bertillon, Francis Galton, and others, as the establishment of a physiognomic code of visual interpretation of the body's signs.[31] Importantly, Sekula warns against constructing an overly unitary model of this visual discourse, and points out that the emergence of this apparatus cannot be reduced to the optical model provided by the camera alone. In keeping with this logic, one might note that many of the static photographic studies of criminals were used to construct a cultural typology of bodily form and appearance, whereas Marey appears to have used photography to drain cultural content from the body surface, and from its static image. Mathew Brady's images, for example, provided a compendium of body types designated likely to be inclined to criminal behavior, thus providing a justification for disciplinary action on people who happened to have particular bodily attributes. But in Marey's study of human physiology described above, the specific form and appearance of the head and body, physical proportion, and physiognomic form—those very elements so crucial to the physiognomic code Sekula describes—are rendered invisible. Any distinguishing details of the man performing for Marey, save his gait, are erased from the picture. We can know neither the skin color nor the shape and form of the features of the man whose movements are tracked in the image. Indeed, the color black, present in the black cloth that covers his skin, renders the body invisible rather than functioning as a visual indicator of racial identity. What, then, supports the argument that Marey's method is in fact a disciplinary technique?

A crucial difference between these static photographic techniques and Marey's is of course the fact that the former were produced with the idea of charting deviance, whereas Marey was interested in establishing a record of a norm. But in the context of this consideration of motion study a more significant difference is that the kind of record Brady and others were constructing was essentially anatomical and hence about static form, while Marey's was physiological and hence about physical transformation. The latter's focus on movement required an elision of those aspects of the body not implicated in duration, motility, and temporality. The technique of still photography so uniquely suited to the record of anatomical form functioned in fundamentally different ways from the technique of serial photography and its record of duration and transformation. Marey effectively reorganized the body to make it embody its own status as an object subject to laws of temporality and duration. By eliminating the factor of depth, for example, Marey was able to render the body an entity characterized by duration and process, a living body whose regulated physiological activity is, as Bernard put it, its "most striking characteristic." Between Brady and Marey we see a shift from the observed and analogically classified body to the experimented upon and digitally ordered body. With the transition from the analogic to the digital and from observation to experimentation, we also see a shift in modes of social regulation. The body once rendered innately deviant is now open to "corrective" physiological regulation and transformation.

Tracking and disciplining the moving body was of course not unique to Marey and the nineteenth century. In *Discipline and Punish*, Foucault describes the Prussian regulations of 1743 that specified the economy of movements to be enacted by the soldier in order to use his time most efficiently: six stages to bring one's weapon to one's foot, four to extend it, thirteen to raise it to the shoulder, and so on. Marey's studies, though conducted more than a century later, were also conducted in large part to gain knowledge about the function of the human body in the military and in sport; to find ways to streamline and capitalize on the energy exerted by the human body in motion; and to make the body conform to physiological standards.

Describing the eighteenth-century military implementation of the body in motion, Foucault states:

> Through this new technique of subjection a new object was being formed; slowly, it superseded the mechanical body—the body composed of solids and assigned movements, the image of which had haunted those who dreamt of disciplinary perfection. This new object is the natural body, the bearer of forces and the seat of duration; the body susceptible to specified operations, which have their order, their stages, their internal conditions, their constituent elements.[32]

This natural body that emerged in the eighteenth century as "the bearer of forces and the seat of duration" is a distinctly living and moving body, and hence a body whose most telling characteristics elude static or death-oriented investigatory techniques such as autopsy or anatomical photography. This temporal and physiological body is further described by Foucault as a system under construction—one that is exercised, manipulated, and trained to perform the work of the state and industry. This industrious body is precisely the body whose functions and processes Marey analyzed in his late-nineteenth-century experiments.[33] Chronophotography functioned as a disciplinary technique, then, insofar as it facilitated the establishment of a productive dynamic economy of the body. By theorizing the physiological forces that drove the body to move, think, and act, Marey contributed to the determination of a more efficient rate of locomotion, or a more effective use of the limbs in the military, in industry, and in athletics. And by inserting the body into an apparatus for its physiological analysis, Marey rendered the natural body an entity that must both incorporate and be incorporated within a self-regulating and self-generating apparatus in order to function to its full capacity as a technology of Western culture.

I may be overstating my case here by considering only the tendency toward the flat and the digital in Marey's work. One could certainly point to counterexamples—for example, his sculptural models of birds in flight. However, even these dimensional objects were perceptually contained and flattened. They were positioned in a series along the perimeter of a disc, set in motion, and viewed through slits in a motion-viewing device, much as serial photographs could be arranged and viewed through a zootrope or a similar viewing device. Another example is his study of birds in flight produced for stereoscopic viewing. However, even these three-dimensional studies relied on linearity, albeit a linearity situated in dimensional space. Attached to the birds was a device for generating a point of light. When the birds flew, the light gave the effect of a linear streak which, when photographed, appeared as a continuous line tracing the movement of the bird in flight. Viewed through a stereoscope, one could see a linear inscription of the path of the bird's flight through three-dimensional space. Frank Gilbreth, known for his industrial time and motion investigations, would later adapt this tech-

nique to the study of human bodies performing surgery and producing manufactured goods. His "chronocyclegraphic" studies were filmed with a motion-picture camera rather than photographed.[34] We see in these films a
temporal and linear trajectory of light that represents the movement of the
hands through space. Here we see a rendering in time and space, but it is a
graphic rendering nonetheless.

Given Marey's interest in flat, graphic inscription as a register of living
movement and duration, it is surprising that he received the Cinématographe with a fair degree of skepticism. In Marey's view, this instrument,
so well suited to the *representation* of movement, presented significant methodological problems in the *analysis* of movement—mainly because the technique of image projection built into the Cinématographe facilitated the
viewing of the filmstrip as a continuous moving image. Marey was interested
in measuring the difference between successive images, a project that was
certainly not furthered by the appearance of continuous movement generated by film projection. The moving image was of little use to his project
precisely because it did not facilitate the analytical and disciplinary task un-
dertaken in chronophotography. Paradoxically, Marey's emphasis on the differential between images—the very factor that would facilitate the sensation
of a continuous moving scene in projection—is the primary element distinguishing chronophotography from cinematography. Whereas the success of
the popular cinema would depend, in part, on the spectatorial sensation of
viewing a continuous moving image and the masking of the technology that
produced this illusion, the physiological cinema would remain committed to
its interest in the representation of duration through a series of static frames,
and to its foregrounding of the apparatus.[35] It is precisely this interest in the
differential between successive still images and the mechanism of movement
analysis that made the quest for a spectatorial cinema a less than fruitful endeavor for Marey. As Adolf Nichtenhauser has pointed out, Marey's *Le mouvement* of 1894 is devoted almost completely to motion recording, leaving
the synthetic reconstruction of movement to a few final pages.[36] Thus it is
not because Marey was unable to imagine a projection apparatus that he
failed to make such an instrument to animate his serial images before his
death; although movement was a central concern to physiologists like
Marey, the spectator's empirical experience of motion and its representation
through film projection were, quite basically, elements at odds with physiology's epistemological project, its desire to measure and to control living
movement.

On whom was the disciplinary power of the chronophotographic apparatus exercised? Earlier in this chapter I described at length the way that the experimental apparatus both pervades and incorporates the body of the analyst
as well as the analyzed subject. I described the action on the body of the
horse effected by Marey and Chauveau's implantation of tambours into its

heart. I also described the horse's body as a mechanism in the apparatus, an element that, quite significantly, triggered and generated the kymograph's inscription device. And I recounted Shaffer's discussion of the body of the astronomical observer as a mechanism incorporated and disciplined within a self-regulating experimental apparatus. In both of these examples, I emphasized the degree to which the body of the observer, and the act of observation itself, was displaced or challenged. In the final section of this chapter, I turn to the work of Marey's students and successors to demonstrate how the Cinématographe figured into the disciplinary techniques of the graphic method. In later chapters, I repeatedly consider what I describe as a particular anxiety on the part of the scientists or technicians—an anxiety about the failure of sensory perception to function autonomously or unproblematically as a means of disciplining and knowing the bodies observed. I argue that the dependency on technology, and the dispersal of embodied sight, triggered in science some often peculiar attempts to maintain authority over subjects by maintaining authority over the optical field. But I also argue that these attempts at centralized corporeal control by technical managers (doctors, technicians, scientists, radiologists) are complicated by the body under study. The living body, as object of technical knowledge, often functioned as a dynamic force within the experimental apparatus, a force that eluded and reflexively disciplined the gaze of the technical observer. As I shall show, this disciplinary action took place not through reflexive observation (a reversal or refusal of the gaze) but through a confounding of the visual logic of observation and appearance.

In what follows I attempt to locate this tendency in the early film motion study, and in a cinematic practice that developed directly out of the work of Marey. In the case that I describe, the body of the test subject is ultimately incorporated as a piece of machinery in an apparatus designed reflexively to test the efficacy and epistemological soundness of the method of physiological time and motion study. Control over instrumental mechanisms and data inscription—those very elements that, by the turn of the century, compounded and even supplanted sensory observation—become a site of instability in the physiological experiment. I shall now examine a case in which the body studied, that of an unconscious animal, is made a part of an apparatus that challenges the capacity of the observer to observe and to know. The experimental subject, like the astral body described by Bernard as so elusive to experimental knowledge, confounds experimental method insofar as its vital characteristics stand outside the range of observational control. Here the animal surrogate for the human body facilitates a fantasy of total corporeal control, while also playing a crucial part in an apparatus that puts observation to an exacting test.

The Cinematic Apparatus in Physiology

By 1900, Marey was the director of an institution devoted to the professional dissemination of physiology as a scientific method, the International Institute for the Control of Instruments and Unification of Methods in Physiology. By 1904, the year of his death, the monumental project of physiology's unification and control had become synonymous with Marey's name; the control of instruments and apparatuses, and not simply bodies, subjects, and communities, had become a central concern of the newly renamed Marey Institute. For Marey's followers, cinematography was not a method in itself, but was one among a range of techniques and instruments potentially to be implemented in the apparatus for the dissemination of physiology as the effort to control not only the living body but the scientific study of life as well.

While a number of scientists and doctors in Europe and North America independently experimented with cinematography as a research technique after 1895, none conducted this kind of research in as systematic a fashion as the physiologists at the Marey Institute and the Collège de France. The cinematic motion studies of Marey's successors make up a unique example of the incorporation of the disciplinary techniques of kymography and chronophotography into the Cinématographe. Through their experiments, cinematic motion study emerged as a methodology rather than as an idiosyncratic or novel scientific technique. Cinematic time and motion study at the Marey Institute and elsewhere in France included analyses of exterior body movement in neurology, studies of microscopic life, and X-ray films of living organisms. Later examples of all of these approaches will be closely considered in subsequent chapters of this book. Notable are the popular films of microscopic life produced by Jean Comandon—footage that gained international recognition through its adoption in the German educational film division of Germany's Ufa (Universumfilm Aktiengesellschaft) and in archives in other countries.[37] Also noteworthy is the work of Lucien Bull, whose studies of ballistics and insect locomotion, along with the work of Comandon and other followers of Marey, belatedly captivated members of the film avant-garde (including Germaine Dulac and Luis Buñuel) after they were exhibited at the Vieux Colombier in 1924.[38] I will return to the popular appropriation of the physiological motion study shortly, after considering more closely the early experiments and their place in the laboratory.

Nichtenhauser notes that the first of Marey's students to use cinematography in motion study in a consistent and exacting manner was Georges Marinesco, a neurologist from Bucharest who studied with both Marey and Charcot (whose serial photography at the Salpêtrière will be considered briefly in the next chapter). In 1898, Marinesco began making films of paraplegics and hemiplegics in order to study their gait.[39] His film work may have been done in conjunction with that of Albert Londe, Charcot's photographer, who also, in consultation with Marey, experimented with cinematic (as well as photographic) motion studies of patients suffering from movement disorders around the turn of the century. In Marinesco's research, cinematography was used in conjunction with a battery of instruments of measurement and documentation. For example, in his research on nerve cells he used the ultramicroscope, a special kind of "darkfield" microscope that diverts light rays and conducts them through particles from the sides rather than only from above, thus illuminating particles without illuminating the field in which they are situated. And as a student at the Salpêtrière, Marinesco used radiography to investigate bone changes in acromegaly, a condition characterized by enlargement of the bones due to hypersecretion of the pituitary hormone.[40] Marinesco's work as a whole demonstrates that, in physiology, cinematography was only one technique among a battery of optical instruments and techniques.

A fairly extensive body of research conducted at the Marey Institute and involving the Cinématographe is the film motion study of Charles-Emile François-Franck, assistant to Marey in the laboratory of pathologic physiology of the Collège de France after 1875, and Marey's successor in the college's chair of physiology. François-Franck's work demonstrates how, in the complex apparatus of the physiological laboratory, the body of the subject experimented upon becomes a crucial site of instability and disruption, though it is subject to intensive management and discipline. In the mid-1880s, François-Franck conducted studies in cerebral circulation and localization of function in conjunction with the neurologist Albert Pitres, who was then working under Charcot at the Salpêtrière.[41] Charcot's work on cerebral localization is cited as the inspiration for this collaboration. The experiments considered below were conducted by François-Franck alone and were part of the research for a book that he would later publish on motor function of the brain—a text for which Charcot wrote the preface.[42]

Marey and Charcot influenced a number of physiologists who worked in film motion study. However, François-Franck's approach to the technique differs in a fundamental way from that of Charcot's photographer Albert Londe to serial photography. Whereas the well-known psychiatric photography of hysteria at the Salpêtrière was conducted in order to establish a typology of outward stages or signs, François-Franck's neurological cinematography was done to provide evidence of the temporal and spatial course of motor transmission within and through the body. In other words, the Salpêtrière photography was an attempt to assign meaning to the progressive external affects of organic and psychogenetic disorders—to classify external movements as specific signs of pathology. François-Franck's stated concern, however, was strictly with organic motor function dissociated from its links to outward expression, emotion, meaning, or health/pathology. Subjectivity and the agency of the subject whose body was being studied were elided from view with his apparent focus on the purely mechanical.

In an essay from 1904 on a photographic analysis technique that he called the "graphocinematographic method," François-Franck describes a film technique that he used to study tendon reflexes in humans and animals. The essay demonstrates how the scientist's stated focus on the purely mechanical is subtended by a desire to regulate and transform the body whose movements are "merely observed." Earlier I argued that the Edison Company's 1903 *Electrocuting an Elephant* reveals a public fascination with execution, and that this fascination was part of a broader scientific fascination with the instrumentation of life and death. Audiences took "scientific" pleasure in the sight of death—a pleasure that involved witnessing the precise moment of death and studying that moment on film again and again. The François-Franck film of animal tendon reflexes, I argue below, demonstrates a similar pleasure—a pleasure in the ritual of torture. Although this film was made in the relative privacy of the laboratory for the eyes of scientists and not for the public, it nonetheless functions as a ceremony of corporal punishment. Foucault, in his discussion of penal institutions, has noted that "the tortured body is first inscribed in the legal ceremonial that must produce, open for all to see, the truth of the crime."[43] In François-Franck's film, the body experimented upon is inscribed in a scientific ritual (the experiment) that must produce, for the scientific eye, the truth of a different elusive entity, "life." Here we find the insensible (chloroformed) animal standing in for the human body. The condemned animal body is made to yield knowledge not about itself but about the hidden and transient processes of "life" that allow other bodies to function as mechanisms in the public sphere (for example, in the industrial workplace, in military service, or in sport). The sacrificial animal body, subjected to physical constraints, pain, and dismemberment, is made to reveal truths not about its own life but about the "purely mechanical" forces that motor "life" in general. What is at stake in the film I describe below, then, is not knowledge about the particular body or species studied, but the scientist's ability to track and discipline the broader life force the experiment embodies—a force that traverses bodies and the technologies that monitor and transform them.

François-Franck details a laboratory procedure involving a comparative study of kymographic and cinematographic recording in the quantitative measurement of physiology.[44] The filmed set was composed as follows. The back leg of a chloroformed dog was held in place within the laboratory setup, the remainder of its body fully hidden from view (covered by a dark cloth). A hammer mounted to a spring was made to strike the unconscious dog's tendon. The jolt triggered the leg, and the movement of the leg intercepted a current, activating an electromagnetic signal transmitted through a wire attached to the Achilles tendon. This signal triggered the inscription of percussion through a myograph (an instrument for recording effects of muscle contraction). A chronometer with a single needle was included in the set to establish a rate of time within each film frame. Finally, a kymograph inscribed a temporal register of the event, stimulated by the vibrations of a tuning fork. The kymographic record appears at the edge of the film frame.

In this experiment, what is ostensibly at issue is the establishment of an accurate measure of reflex speed. In other words, François-Franck was after an accurate means of measuring bodily movement, and not most significantly a measurement of movement in the particular body in question. The complexity of the apparatus alone should give some indication of the difficulties in devising a measurement apparatus and establishing its accuracy. The filmstrip served as a visual record of the means of measurement, which included a clock, a kymographic record, and two graphic inscription devices. Like the astronomical observatory's director who, in Shaffer's account, checked and calibrated his observer's performance against the data he obtained from the chronoscope, François-Franck was able to check and calibrate the performance of the kymograph, the clock, and the cinema film against one another. François-Franck's apparatus might be compared to the process of the gaze, which never directly appropriates its object but must pass through a series of relays. But this apparatus ultimately displaces the gaze altogether by forcing it to pass through a series of checkpoints that displace the image with graphical data. François-Franck's experiment is perhaps in part about rendering docile and compliant the body of the dog as a substitute for the human body. It is also about checking and calibrating the viability and accuracy of observation within the terms of the experimental apparatus; the agent of this performance, however, is quite different from the agent whose performance is calibrated in Shaffer's observatory. Here we find that agency is dispersed throughout the heterogeneous elements of the apparatus, resting in the kymograph, the clock, and the film image, as well as in the bodies of the observer and the observed. It is the apparatus that is put to the test, and not the body of the observer alone.

The brief cinematographic record of this dog's reflex action functions simultaneously as pictorial and graphic record. Pictorially, the film shows the leg being struck by the hammer and its subsequent rise, fall, and return to stasis. The film functions also as a pictorial record of the kymographic register in production. It shows the inscription of the two graphical lines, one charting the striking of the hammer, the other the movement of the leg. The cinema film thus serves as a control image as well as a temporal gauge in itself. Although the camera is, by necessity, the only instrument out of frame, its presence is later signified by the film frames reproduced in François-Franck's essay with sprocket holes visible (figures 2.7 and 2.8). His essay's frame-by-frame analysis not only considers the differences between film images but

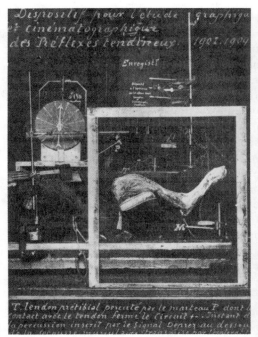

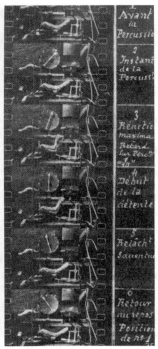

Figure 2.7. Engraving of laboratory setup as it appears in Charles-Emile François-Franck, "Application de la méthode graphotographique . . . ," *Comptes rendus de la Société de biologie* 2 (1904).

Figure 2.8. Frame enlargements and text as they appear in François-Franck, "Application de la méthode grapho-photographique."

also compares the film image data with every register of representation operating in the apparatus.

Earlier I posed the question, On whom is the disciplinary power of the chronophotographic apparatus exercised? I have attempted to demonstrate, through the example of François-Franck's graphocinematographic apparatus, that disciplinary power is exercised both on and through the apparatus, a system that incorporates the bodies of the observer and the observed, dispersing agency across technologies and bodies. But what role does the body of the observed play in this system? I also suggested that, in the case of François-Franck's experiment, the body of the test animal complicates the experimental system, confounding efforts to derive a standardized, reliable source of scientific knowledge. This claim may appear difficult to support: the body in question is that of an unconscious dog. But what is at issue, of course, is not only the dog's willful resistance, but the overall success or failure of the experiment to render visible this animal's submission to the disciplining apparatus.

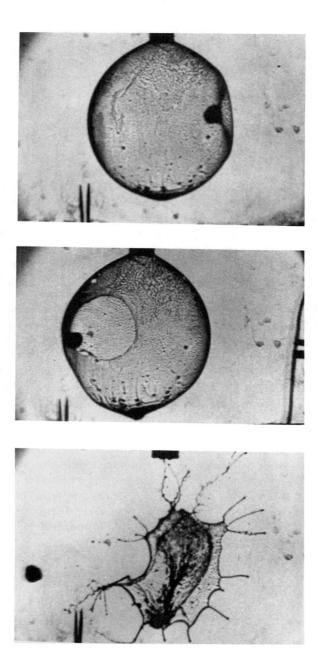

Figure 2.9. Frames from Lucien Bull's 1904 film motion study of a bullet penetrating a soap bubble.

A second example may help to clarify the metaphorical implications of this experiment: the physiologist Lucien Bull's 1904 production at the Marey Institute of a slow-motion cinematic film of a bullet penetrating a soap bubble.[45] Bull altered a movie camera, removing its lens and rebuilding its interior to construct a stereoscopic slow-motion system that could take more than two thousand images per second. A sprocketless roll of film fifty-four images in length was wrapped around the drum of the camera and exposed by the illumination of an electric spark that flared intermittently (every two-thousandth of a second). The film Bull produced was projected at a normal rate, slowing the imperceptible moment of the bullet's bursting of the bubble to a speed at which it could be perceived and analyzed. In this example, the imperceptible moment of the soap bubble's figurative death is rendered visible (figure 2.9). It can be analyzed, frame by frame. This film functions like a metaphorical rendering of Bernard's experiments of destruction, the soap bubble standing in for the experimental subject as the source of life that must be intercepted and severed in order to be studied and known. Here we have an "experiment" that succinctly demonstrates the relationship between visuality and destruction inherent in the experimental process.

It is finally Edison's *Electrocuting an Elephant* that best demonstrates the place of "scientific" looking in public culture. The film preceded François-Franck's by only a year. The popular Edison reel bears a critical likeness to François-Franck's physiological study not only because it documents an extreme intervention in the living processes of a test subject but also because it reflexively documents the complex place that technologies of representation had come to occupy in the regulation and control of life and death. Here we see science experiment as popular cultural ritual. But I would argue that the ritual is a means not only of punishing the "wild beast" for its noncompliance with modern Western modes of entertainment culture, but of carrying out a fantasy of discipline and corporal punishment through observation—an exercise of disciplinary authority through sight that is no longer viable by the turn of the century. As we shall see in subsequent chapters, scientists' attempt to observe, document, and measure the physiological systems of the body were continually confounded by the forces of the body that the film motion study set out to trace and to destroy.

CHAPTER 3

An Etiology of the
Neurological Gaze

FOUCAULT HAS SHOWN THAT the institution of pathological anatomy entailed a shift in focus from symptoms to organs, sites, and causes. With the rise of physiology later in the century, the body was reconfigured as a system, a network of functions taking place across organs and sites. Viewing the body and its parts as static entities and reading its surface alone were no longer viable methods of determining pathology. Of what use, then, were conventional body images—representations of the surface of the body? Certainly they have not dropped out of medical practice. Their persistence is more than evident in the example of videotelemetry, a technique currently used experimentally in neurology to monitor epileptics. The patient lying in bed is hooked up to an electroencephalograph machine and placed before a video camera. The camera is left on around the clock, its continuous image available at any time for comparison with the simultaneously generated electroencephalogram. Clearly, surveillance of the body continues to be an important technique in medical practice.

In this chapter, I attempt to historicize the contemporary neurological inscription of the body by considering some of the uses of the film motion study in the field of neurology. The nineteenth-century neurological motion study has been the topic of extensive feminist analysis.[1] A number of important studies have addressed the work of neurologist Jean-Martin Charcot. A practitioner championing the empirical techniques characteristic of nineteenth-century neurology, Charcot is most often presented as the figure against whom Freud reacted in his construction of the new science of psychoanalysis, and a figure whose practice marked the close of an era of psychiatric imaging. However, it is important to recall that neurology did not die out with the rise of psychoanalysis and the talking cure in the twentieth century. Neurological researchers and clinicians, though plagued by the limitations of empirical looking and the implicit challenge posed by newer ways of conceptualizing and imaging mental illness, continued to read the body's surface for signs of pathology. Psychoanalysis did not so much correct or supersede neurology as supplement it, if in contradictory ways, providing a more focused subspecialty in the treatment of mental illness. The visual techniques associated with neurology that persisted throughout the period in which psychoanalysis became institutionalized thus deserve consideration as a set of practices complicit with psychoanalysis in the twentieth-century medical management of mental illness.

I focus on neurology for another important reason: it is impossible to discuss films produced in neurology during the first half of this century without raising questions about scientific spectatorship, visual pleasure, and cinematic surveillance. Neurologists clearly were fascinated by images of the body out of control. Such images were analyzed in the relative privacy of the laboratory and clinic or in the context of the medical professional meeting. Motion studies were viewed closely and repeatedly, whether through loop projection of films at scientific gatherings or through frame analyses conducted in the laboratory and published in professional journals. What was the neurologist's professional stake in subjecting patients to this kind of optical scrutiny? Many of the films that are considered below document conditions that clearly caused patients great somatic and psychical pain. These people are in most cases filmed nude or nearly nude and while unconscious or performing movements involuntarily. Patient identity and agency become crucial issues in the face of a form of documentation that so drastically reduces the person imaged to a cipher of physiological perversion and graphic unintelligibility. It is just this perverse unintelligibility, I will suggest, that subverts the surveillant neurological gaze. Fascinated by the unnatural rhythms and incomprehensible sequences of movement displayed by patients, the neurologists considered in this chapter were ultimately forced to confront the impossibility of controlling the disorderly bodies that populated their field of vision.

The example of neurological motion study familiar to most readers is the serial photography of hysterics produced by Désiré Magloire and Paul Regnard, interns working under Charcot at the Paris Salpêtrière asylum, and Albert Londe, a chemist hired as asylum photographer by Charcot, in the middle to late nineteenth century. Using techniques similar to those employed by Marey and Muybridge, these men produced serial photographs to analyze the movements associated with hysteria. A fact less familiar to most readers, however, is that Charcot was also involved in the analysis of a wide range of nervous system pathologies (including tabes dorsalis, multiple sclerosis, poliomyelitis, and Tourette syndrome). Londe, in consultation with Marey, made serial motion studies for analysis not only of hysteria but also of other types of movement disorders associated with organic illness (figure 3.1). Although these images have not been as broadly studied as the serial photographs of hysteria that were reproduced in the asylum's two publications, the *Iconographie photographique de la Salpêtrière* (1870–80) and the

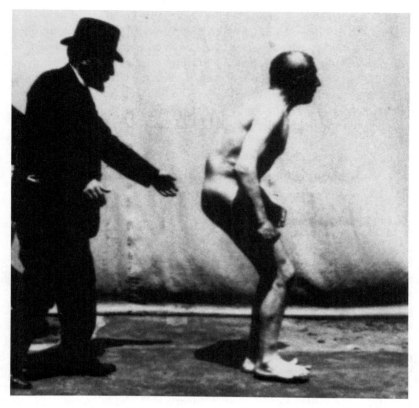

Figure 3.1. Frame from one of Albert Londe's chronophotographic series for analysis of pathological movement.

Nouvelle iconographie de la Salpêtrière (1888-1918), they nonetheless suggest that the scope of visual analysis at that institution extended beyond Charcot and beyond hysteria.

In what follows, I begin with a brief consideration of some of the critical writings on the Salpêtrière photographic studies of hysteria. I do this not because I want to take issue with the arguments put forward in these essays, but because this work, which is on some level about the origins of psychoanalysis, sets up a critical framework that in effect makes difficult a consideration of the status of neurology and the perception of organic illness during the period that psychoanalysis came to prominence. This chapter takes as its subject, then, the techniques and methods of neurology that persisted throughout the first half of the twentieth century.

Empiricism and Visuality in Neurology

In 1978, Jacqueline Rose reminded her readers that Freud's work on hysteria started with a rejection of Charcot's "simple mapping of symptoms onto the body."[2] Psychoanalysis rejected neurology's regard of the clinical signs of hysteria as self-evidence of genetically inherent organic disease. "The problem with Charcot's work," Rose explained, "is that while he was constructing the symptomatology of the disease . . . he was reinforcing [hysteria] as a special category of behavior, visible to the eye and the result of a degenerate hereditary disposition."[3] The problem to which Rose referred is Charcot's part in what Foucault has called "the great degenerescence system" that supported eugenics and racist science.[4] Foucault explained that

> psychoanalysis was established in opposition to a certain kind of psychiatry, the psychiatry of degeneracy, eugenics and heredity. . . . Indeed, in relation to that psychiatry—which is still the psychiatry of today's psychiatrists—psychoanalysis played a liberating role.[5]

Like Foucault, Rose emphasized the role psychoanalysis played in the rejection of the biologism that grounded this neurologically based psychiatry—a rejection especially of psychiatry's insistence on a biologically based system for organizing and ranking bodies according to categories such as intelligence, class, race, gender, and sexuality. Rose also emphasized the importance of visual and empirical techniques in this system. Her account suggests that psychoanalysis implicitly rejected visuality and empiricism when it opposed Charcot's essentialist biologism, and that this move entailed a shift in the ranking of the senses. Significantly, Freud challenged Charcot's methods specifically by developing techniques based in speech and hearing. Consequently, by the mid-twentieth century, sight and the body's surface appearance would no longer be regarded as reliable indicators of mental pathology; speech and audition would overtake them in the sensory hierarchy of psychoanalysis. As Rose summarized, "it was only in penetrating behind the visible symptom of a disorder and asking what it was the symptom was trying to *say*" that Freud could challenge Charcot's empiricist and biologistic formulation of hysteria.[6]

Rose notes that Freud's break with Charcot's empiricism entailed a questioning of neurology's reliance on the clinical photograph as evidence of organic pathology. Her argument takes as a given the idea that images (and sight) are aligned with empiricist and biologistic methods at the turn of the century. In his analysis of the photographic documentation of mental illness, Sander Gilman makes a similar point: "Freud rejected the idea of seeing the patient, thus centering psychoanalysis on the process of listening"; and "in rejecting the rigid representationalism of nineteenth-century theories of understanding mental processes, Freud also rejected their basis of empirical proof."[7] Although Rose and Gilman offer very different analyses, they share the view that the empiricism Freud rejected was crucially dependent on visual modes of knowledge. In addition, they suggest that speech and hearing were historically more subtle and humane analytical techniques that implicitly challenged the empirical techniques of racist science—techniques that would come to their fullest expression in Nazi science and medicine.[8] For Gilman, Charcot's visual methods lacked the sensitivity and specificity of techniques used in the talking cure. He quotes a passage from Theodor Reik in which the orthodox follower of Freud stresses the importance of auditory techniques. Reik describes what he calls "the third ear," which, he suggests, the analyst must use to decode the asides that are "whispered between sentences" and pick up "what is said pianissimo" in the course of the analysis.

Gilman's account suggests that the Salpêtrière photographs can be regarded as a part of a broader set of typological systems introduced in the Enlightenment and developed throughout the eighteenth and nineteenth centuries (including, for example, anthropometry, craniometry, and phrenology). As Nancy Leys Stepan has shown, these sciences encoded the anatomy and physical appearance of primarily non-Europeans and, later, European women, as indicators of a lower developmental or evolutionary state.[9] These practices relied heavily on the ranking of visually apparent physical characteristics according to supposed capacity for intelligence, motor skill, and so on. Rose points out that psychoanalysis challenged this type of biologistic and empirical pathologizing of sexualized bodies. The radical moment of this intervention, she explains, was when Freud began to question the normalizing force of psychiatric techniques—the field's establishment of a ranked hierarchy of intelligence, health, and morality tied to categories of gender, race, and class. Freud's intervention was specifically in relation to sexuality, questioning "the social definition of sexual perversion as 'innate' or 'degenerate.'"[10] Freud's break with "the great degenerescence system" was thus, for Rose, Gilman, and other writers, critically linked to a break both with visual techniques of analysis and psychiatry's labeling of sexual practices outside of those established as heterosexual norms as pathological.

Although the depathologization of homosexual behavior in Freud's work was without question a radical moment in the history of psychiatry, it is important to note that visuality nonetheless survived its association with empiricism. Indeed, visuality has emerged at the center of a vast medical industry and subspecialty encompassing a plethora of postempirical imaging techniques.[11] And though Freud's work posed a crucial challenge to theories of sexuality that posit homosexuality as a pathological condition and heterosexuality as a norm, it has also been used to support institutional efforts to reinforce norms of sexual conduct. I would ask, then, with Foucault, "why this sacralising modesty that insists on denying that psychoanalysis has anything to do with normalization?"[12] If, as Foucault has argued, many of today's psychiatrists still practice the neurologically informed psychiatry of degeneracy, eugenics, and heredity, they do so in part because comparatively little has been done to transform the understanding of the designation of organic pathology, and to unpack the meanings of the category of the biological. Although psychoanalysis provided a method for recognizing the historical and cultural basis of behavior—that deemed normal as well as that deemed pathological—it ultimately did not fully challenge or preclude neurology's authority in the conceptualization and treatment of disorders and diseases with designated links to organic sources. Distinguishing among organic, psychogenic, and social causes of behavior has been as much a matter of divvying up bodies among professional territories as uncovering the "true" source of pathological behavior.

Because this chapter focuses primarily on techniques for managing disorders understood to be organically based, the view of psychoanalysis as a more humane or progressive methodology deserves further consideration. By proving the viability of psychoanalytic explanation and nonorganic etiologies, psychoanalysis has without question challenged the normalizing and disciplining force of neurology. However, in some instances the insistence on a psychogenic etiology has proved as debilitating as the insistence on genetic and organic explanations that we see in Charcot's work on women hysterics, or in psychiatry's designation of homosexuality as a pathological condition.

A case in point is the treatment of Tourette syndrome (TS), an underdiagnosed disorder first reported in the nineteenth century and sometimes referred to as "male hysteria." Observed by both Charcot and Freud, Tourette syndrome was named after one of its principal researchers, Gilles de la Tourette, who was a student of Charcot. As with hysteria and other mental illnesses, the etiology of TS was attributed to neuropathic heredity by its early investigators. However, by the turn of the century, it was more common to see it attributed to degeneracy and mental instability. As neurology moved toward an understanding of psychogenic factors in mental pathology, and as psychoanalysis gained ground, psychological factors were privileged over possible organic causation in the search for an etiology. Exhibiting a variety of symptoms shared by pathologies attributed to psychological causes (symptoms such as motor and phonic tics, involuntary utterances, impulsive ideas, and obsessive-compulsive behavior), TS was assumed to be a psychogenic disorder and, from about 1920 until the late 1960s, it was treated with therapies designed to uncover a psychical trauma. However, current research on TS favors its categorization as a genetically transmitted disorder.

One could certainly argue that genetic etiologies are bound to predominate in research on many diseases in an era (the 1990s) designated by the American Psychiatric Association as "the decade of the brain." However, the emphasis on psychogenic etiologies that predominated in TS research for forty years deserves critical consideration also. The insistence on a psychogenic etiology in the face of evidence of possible organic factors is perplexing. Here one is reminded of Gilles Deleuze and Félix Guattari's critique of psychoanalysis for making a universal dogma of the Oedipal narrative, and for inducing the patient to conform to this dogma in the course of treatment.[13] Similarly, the progress of TS research has been driven in part by the desire to strengthen psychoanalysis as an institution and by the need to carve out the respective territories of psychoanalysis and neurology by distinguishing between social and organic factors, as if the two could be separated. The relatively recent finding that TS has a very strong organic component has made it clear in retrospect that clinical insistence on psychological factors was, in this instance, as politically retrograde and culturally stigmatizing as Charcot's insistence on hereditary and organic etiologies was in the treatment of hysteria.

Here I want to consider the link between perversion and pathology in order to further consider the significance of the split between the organic and the psychogenic, and between neurology and psychoanalysis. Organic pathology functions culturally, somewhat like the notion of perversion, by subverting the logic of normativity inscribed in physical acts. Kaja Silverman notes that Janine Chasseguet-Smirgel's reading of perversion "suggests that its significance extends far beyond the domain of the purely sexual."[14] I quote from Silverman:

> The theoretical interest of perversion extends even beyond the disruptive force it brings to bear upon gender. It strips sexuality of all functionality, whether biological or social; in an even more extreme fashion than "normal" sexuality, it puts the body and the world of objects to uses that have nothing whatever to do with any immanent design or purpose.[15]

Silverman explains that perversion has a broad social function, turning aside "not only from hierarchy and genital sexuality, but from the paternal signifier."[16] I want to suggest a use of the concept of perversion here to analyze the regard of activities overdetermined by organic factors. This use of the concept is justified in part by the fact that designated pathological movement associated with organic illness is often interpreted by its observers as a sign of perversion. Just as sexual perversion strips sexuality of functionality, putting the body to uses that have nothing to do with immanent purpose, so the involuntary tics, tremors, or seizures of patients living with organic disease strip movement of its functionality. The pathological body engages in acts that have nothing to do with purpose. However, the aberrant behavior of the person with organically based pathology is driven not only by the unconscious but by organic processes that organize the movements of the body in ways that often are later encoded as perverse by scientific and lay spectators. If, as Silverman notes, sexual perversion is always organized to some degree by what it subverts (Oedipus), then neurologically induced behavior also may be organized by what *it* subverts, namely, the apparent order and logic of meaningful, expressive movement. And if, as Silverman also notes, the practices associated with sexual perversion subvert the binary oppositions that support the social order (as necrophilia subverts the life/death dichotomy, or as masochism subverts the pleasure/pain distinction), then somatic actions associated with organic pathology challenge the binary oppositions that support the order of mental health: the distinctions of organic/psychogenic, health/illness, voluntary/involuntary activity.

My point is not, of course, that organic illness escapes social determinants, but that it introduces a level of somatic determination beyond the particular factors that organize the unconscious, inserting into the social a degree of disorder that is difficult to contain within an Oedipal narrative. Yet it is almost always the neurologist's wont to inscribe the patient's arbitrary behavior into such a narrative. I am interested here in this drive to organize organically based symptoms around an Oedipal narrative and in the ways in which the patient's actions elude or subvert that narrative process. Involuntary movements and impulsive phonic utterances are, in effect, limit cases, signifying for those who witness them a living death of control over meaning. I return to my example of Tourette syndrome to clarify this point. The involuntary curses, barks, tics, expressed thoughts, and compulsions of the person with TS cannot be attributed to an original psychical trauma or event. Nevertheless, the symptoms themselves insistently invoke the paternal signifier for their observers—that is, in some instances they are viewed by the medical community and the general public alike as perverse behavior, an exhibition that has meaning only in terms of a narrative of excess and perversion. The fact that these expressions or actions are involuntary and without direction (they are not directed to a particular person or group) does little to dispel the assignment of a narrative of transgression. People with TS are consistently labeled evil, delinquent, rude, and so on. The cultural logic that retroactively contains their involuntary actions maintains the institutional grounds of neurology and psychiatry.

In the pages that follow, I consider two sets of films in order to argue that the perverse movements symptomatic of organic illness subvert neurology's social order. The patients who perform these movements act as agents in this process; however, that agency is not always wholly determined by will or the forces of the patient's unconscious but is a collective process of multiple causality enacted through the body. I will argue that by short-circuiting the pathways of the patient's individual subjective experience, of the unconscious, and of expression, organic disease functions as a wrench in the signifying practices that organize subjectivity, identity, and social order as they are perceived by the neurological observer. At the very least, the symptoms of organic pathology undermine neurology's logic of appearances and its modes of visual knowledge.

The first set of films I consider is a group of short studies of convulsive seizures produced in 1905 at a New York State public institution for epileptics. In this project, the motion picture camera was used to supplement surveillance measures already in place at the institution. However, cinematography proved a less than adequate instrument for the task of charting the interior physiology of epilepsy. Not long after Marey's foundational work in physiological motion study—and his rejection of the cinema—these neurologists questioned the motion picture's ability to represent adequately what was regarded as the most significant aspect of epilepsy's physiology: its status as a chemically and electrically based process acting at the margins of the perceptual field. Although the motion picture camera prosthetically augmented institutional surveillance of the epileptic seizure, its images offered very little toward a modern etiology of epilepsy, much less toward prognosis and cure. Rather, cinematography proved to be a technique for imputing meaning to the movements of bodies out of control. Epilepsy repeatedly confounded neurologists' attempts to regulate disorderly bodies and construct a clear etiologic narrative.

The second group of films I consider was produced between 1918 and the end of World War II. Designated a "cinematographic atlas" of nervous diseases, these films were made by New York neurophysiologists to document mental diseases. The atlas revives some of the visual conventions of classification and typology used a century earlier in physiognomy and pathological anatomy; in doing so, it raises important questions for psychoanalytic feminist critiques of visuality. The atlas makes use of these earlier conventions not to regenerate empirical techniques of nineteenth-century neurology, but to support case analyses that are informed by the postempirical science of psychoanalysis. I argue that these conventions were resuscitated partly to ease professional anxieties about the declining status of sight-based diagnosis. If film could not be used to control disease and to construct an etiology, it could at least be used to model "classical" signs of disease for medical students and doctors. But modeled in these films is also the neurologist's own confounded attempts to contain organic pathology in a coherent narrative. In a sense, these films drew on the visual techniques of nineteenth-century neurology in order to contain new and complex manifestations of mental disease within a familiar historical framework. They created an image of timeless institutional knowledge of pathologies at a time when neurology was faced with epidemic encephalitis, a disease that repeatedly confounded neurological investigation by exhibiting symptoms typical of psychopathologies. Though film images sometimes helped neurologists more accurately to distinguish among the clinical signs of psychopathology and organic pathology, they were of little use in determining the etiology, long-term prognosis, and treatment of certain diseases—particularly those with organic components, such as encephalitis (viral inflammation of the brain). As Oliver Sacks points out, encephalitis lethargica (sleeping sickness) and Tourette syndrome both virtually disappeared from clinical studies for decades during this century, not for lack of patients, but because both disorders were regarded as "strange beyond belief" and "could not be accommodated in the conventional frameworks" of neurological knowledge during the heyday of psychoanalysis.[17] The cinematographic atlas, then, is a stunningly grim compendium of etiologically obscure diseases regarded as "strange beyond belief" because they confound disciplinary norms. Further, it is a vivid document of U.S. neurology's sensory crisis in the face of organic mental disease, as well as of the discipline's own neurotic insistence on the structuring force of paternal law in the expression of mental pathology. In this film atlas, visuality and the biological body converge, decades after Charcot's iconographies; but they appear in a postempirical psychiatric configuration of degeneracy, eugenics, and heredity.

The Epilepsy Biographs

Just after the turn of the century, William Spratling, medical superintendent at the Craig Colony for Epileptics in rural upstate New York, wrote to the American Mutoscope and Biograph Company requesting information on the production of motion pictures. He wanted to document on film his patients' seizures. When in 1905 Walter Greenough Chase, a Boston neurologist, approached the Biograph Company with the same idea, he was placed in contact with Spratling.[18] In the summer of 1905, Chase filmed twenty-one epileptic seizures at the Craig Colony under Spratling's supervision.[19] As the only complete cinematic case study of mental disease intact from this period, these films are a useful text for a reading of the gaze in turn-of-the-century U.S. neurology.

The Craig Colony was a public institution overseen by the New York State Board of Charities. The subjects appearing in what Chase called his "epilepsy biographs" were charges of the state who labored for their keep on the colony farm. It is a prime example of an institution designed to provide both an enclosed space amenable to surveillance and an open space providing the light, ventilation, and physical exertion thought necessary to avoid undue contact, contagion, and overcrowding. As Foucault points out, physicians were among the first managers of collective space, and the institution of public health standards was chiefly a matter of ordering the space of habitation.[20] In contrast to the eighteenth- and nineteenth-century asylum, the colony provided light, open space, entertainment, and a semblance of "normal," mixed-gender community life still lacking in many private and state-run institutions of the period.

The colony was also quite a lucrative investment for the state. In the year that Chase shot the epilepsy biographs, the state cleared a profit from its agricultural and industrial production. That time was provided in the schedule of colony workers to produce the epilepsy biographs suggests that the desire to capture the epileptic seizure on film overrode the demand for productivity. Despite the colony's emphasis on labor and profit, Spratling put at Chase's disposal over one hundred male patients and the colony's entire medical staff. Spratling wrote that Chase's films would aid in prognosis and be useful educational tools. Prognosis alone was a formidable task in the treatment of epilepsy, a disease whose progression was difficult to track, and which is even now a very broadly defined disorder, incorporating a range of diverse symptoms.[21] Although the films may have served as instructional aids in professional lectures, the definition of epilepsy that emerges in Spratling and Chase's accounts suggests that they would have regarded motion study as an unlikely prognostic indicator. A review of Spratling's writings and institutional policies suggests that in fact the films were a part of a larger multifaceted program of surveillance—a program that included monitoring of every aspect of the colony residents' lives, including their routine daily activities, their seizures, and even their anatomical status after death. In what follows, I consider the place of the film study among the battery of surveillance techniques operating at the colony at the turn of the century. However, what emerges from this account is an image of the epileptic body's structural resistance within this particular disciplinary technique.

Foucault notes that autopsy was an important technique in nineteenth-century medicine because it provided the researcher with the opportunity to analyze the interior body. In 1905, the Craig Colony took an active interest in autopsy as a means of pathological analysis. At about the time that Spratling contacted the Biograph Company about filming his patients, a state law was passed granting the Craig Colony the right to perform autopsies on the brains of patients who had died at the institution. Autopsies could now be performed without a patient's prior consent. That from among the numerous institutions in the state of New York, the Craig Colony alone was granted this right, suggests that Spratling was the primary petitioner for the law. "Such a law as this," he claimed, "will aid in the elucidation of the problems underlying the etiology of *the strangest disease in human history*, and every public institution in the State should have a similar one."[22]

The autopsy law guaranteed Spratling a supply of fresh bodies for neurological research—a free reserve guaranteed by his charges' dependency on the state. The factors of destitution and free labor cannot be overlooked in considering Spratling's regard of his living charges as a stock of potential cadavers. Leslie Camhi has emphasized the significance of the fact that

Charcot's first neurological discovery was based on the body of his servant, a sclerotic charwoman whom he hired as a household domestic in order to secure her body for autopsy after death. Charcot's investment paid off, Camhi notes, when he was able to prove his diagnosis in autopsy.[23] Spratling's enthusiasm for the autopsy law suggests that he too looked upon his unpaid laborers with a certain keen anticipation. However, Spratling did not wait for autopsy to analyze his patients optically. He dissected their every movement during life, through a close documentation of their daily routines, and through cinematic frame analysis of their movements during seizures. The autopsy was thus by the turn of the century an ancillary technique, augmenting data from other modes of instrumentation.

Spratling wrote that "so far as possible we record every epileptic seizure that occurs at the colony. All persons employed in the care of patients instantly note every seizure at the moment of its occurrence, writing down the exact hour, the type of seizure and its duration."[24] But his techniques for tracking and recording the conduct of his patients did not operate at all smoothly. Some patients had several hundred seizures a day, making surveillance and recording a monumental task for colony staff. The system was further confounded by the fact that the Colony residents worked throughout many acres of farmland, woods, and buildings—an impossibly vast area for the small staff to monitor thoroughly. Not only did patients have seizures so subtle as to go unseen, they had them in out-of-the-way places, hidden from the tracking gaze of the staff. Colony staff thus was required to occupy the space of residents, trailing them during their most rudimentary bodily tasks, and scrutinizing their most subtle movements and expressions.

The motion picture camera presented itself as a tool able to extend the domain of a surveillant gaze that was already in place at the colony before Chase's arrival in 1905. But Chase and Spratling soon found that cinematic surveillance faced the same obstacles as daily observation by staff. While Chase was bound to a stationary camera and a fixed outdoor set (recall that this is 1905), his potential subjects conducted their daily lives—and their seizures—across the vast complex of the colony. As Chase explains,

> The most difficult pathological movement to reproduce is that of an epileptic seizure, for the reason that . . . your patient is not always so obliging as to have his seizure out of doors in an available place and also at a time when the sun is at its best. . . . The only place successfully to do such work is where there is an abundance of material, as in an epileptic colony.[25]

To increase the likelihood of a seizure's occurrence within range of the camera, Spratling retained very large groups of male patients close by the set at all times. He engaged the colony's medical staff in close and constant watch over this group, so that a body might be lifted up and delivered directly to the camera at the first sign of a seizure. I quote again from Chase's account:

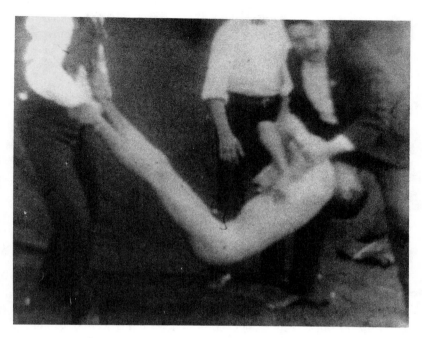

Figure 3.2. Frame from the epilepsy biographs, Walter Greenough Chase (1905).

> Realizing that it was impossible to set up the camera after the seizure had com-
> menced, we had some one hundred and twenty-five male patients from the in-
> firmary assembled in a convenient spot out of doors on a warm summer day.
> The clothes were removed and the patients covered with blankets, so that, a
> seizure occurring, the blanket could be readily dropped and the subject, within a
> very few seconds, placed in the range of the camera.[26]

Chase was interested in capturing on film only the most dramatic moments
of the seizure. In most cases, the men were filmed nude, lying on the ground
outdoors before a dark cloth backdrop or a plain brick wall—a staging remi-
niscent of the sparse clinical sets favored by Marey and Muybridge. As the patient writhed on the ground, the camera, which Chase equipped with a
traveling head, attempted to keep his body in frame. Occasionally caught in
the frame's periphery is a white-coated attendant or a physician in a suit.
Chase apparently turned the camera off during lulls in activity or when the
body wriggled out of the camera's range, in effect editing together in camera
what he regarded as key moments in the seizure. At the head and tail of each
of these short takes, attendants and doctors are briefly visible struggling to de-
liver, remove, or position a body in range of the camera's view (figure 3.2).
Chase did not want to record only the most active moments of seizures;

he was also interested in capturing movements over which patients apparently exerted the least amount of conscious control. As another neurologist-filmmaker of this period put it, "to make the patient perform unconsciously"—that is, to draw out a display of involuntary movement—was a central task of the neurological film director.[27] What was behind this seemingly contradictory idea of commanding the performance of a spontaneous seizure? Chase credits Francis X. Dercum, a neurologist who collaborated with Muybridge, for inspiring his project. Dercum mechanically induced seizures in his experimental subjects. He hired a woman, an artists' model, to pose nude, maintaining a restrictive position for so long that she experienced violent, spasmodic muscular contractions resembling seizure. At the moment the contractions began, Muybridge activated his battery of cameras. Dercum was present at a professional meeting where Chase showed his films. Dercum described this project to the audience there as follows:

> The pictures . . . show the phases of an epileptic seizure. . . . Convulsions were artificially induced by the method described by A. J. Parker and myself at that time, that of muscular excitation with the subject in hypnosis. The convulsions introduced artificially were as genuine as any form of convulsive movement and there was no simulation on the part of the subject.[28]

This insistence that "convulsions introduced artificially were as genuine as any form of convulsive movement" is important because it suggests that Dercum saw no real difference between convulsions caused by organic or psychological factors and those generated by mechanical stimulus. Here the role of the experimenter in the pathological action studied is explicitly acknowledged. As in Bernard's experiments of destruction, the researcher inserts himself in the experimental process by inducing a response. This practice can be traced back to the photographic studies of human expression conducted by Guillaume Benjamin Duchenne (Duchenne de Boulogne), a close associate of Charcot. A project of Duchenne's provides another useful point of reference.

A researcher who worked under Charcot's sponsorship at the Salpêtrière with no official academic chair or hospital appointment, Duchenne is well known for his early description of muscular dystrophy and his research on the physiology of neuropathological movement, which included the development of galvanotherapy, a technique wherein electrical current was applied, ostensibly therapeutically, to people diagnosed with nervous disorders. Part of this project involved photography. Duchenne had an actor mime expressions associated with particular emotions (pain, happiness, and so on) and then applied electrical stimulation to the various muscles of another subject's face until an identical expression was induced there. In this manner, he hoped to identify the distinct muscles engaged in the expression of particular emotions.

Duchenne's experiment played upon an ambiguity about the term "expression," which can imply a look that one wears passively and without intended meaning, or a willful act of signification—the subtle difference between wearing a look upon one's face and casting a look. As Gilman notes, the use of an actor as a prototype for expressions of emotion or sensation is highly problematic because it assumes that an induced performance of a seizure can provide information about spontaneous seizure. I would suggest, though, that what is problematic is not only Duchenne's apparent failure to recognize the inauthenticity of mimed or mechanically induced expression, but also his involvement in the production of "expression." Taking quite literally the agenda of the neurologist who hopes to "make the patient perform unconsciously" for the camera, Duchenne used mechanical induction to force the subject to emit signs of a pathological condition from which she did not in fact suffer. Short-circuiting their subjects' control over their own movements, Duchenne and Dercum both intervened in the life of the subjects they studied in extreme ways. In these examples, the process of imaging the subject is implicated in a blatantly disciplinary act that involves little actual physical intervention. In the case of Dercum's experiment especially, the force exerted upon the body of the women studied is quite obliquely administered.

Although Duchenne presented his project as a visual compendium of typical expressions of living emotion, he in fact produced in his subjects the experience typical only of such people as the Salpêtrière patients—that is, the experience of being unable to exercise control over one's facial configurations and bodily movements. He generated in his subjects the sensory experience of emitting involuntarily a series of motor actions. Duchenne's flagrantly disciplinary action upon the body is indicative of a broader anxiety among neurologists about motor control and normative movement. The way that their subject submitted so easily to mechanical forces suggests that self-control was not guaranteed even among "healthy" subjects. But more importantly, the experiment demonstrated the ease with which the healthy body could be made to mimic pathological expression.

The implications of mimed pathological expression for medical and cultural knowledge are exemplified best by the numerous medicolegal cases of trauma ostensibly caused by industrial technologies (train mishaps and farm and factory machinery accidents, for example). Around 1900, the impact of industrial workplace technologies on the nervous system became a major issue in medicine, law, and industry. Workplace and railway trauma generated extensive legal and medical debates. The numerous claims against companies led industrialists to question the authenticity of the charges that were made against them. For example, the neurologist Allan McLane Hamilton, at the bidding of law firms, analyzed cases in which workers sought compensation for neural and motor impairments that they claimed were the result of

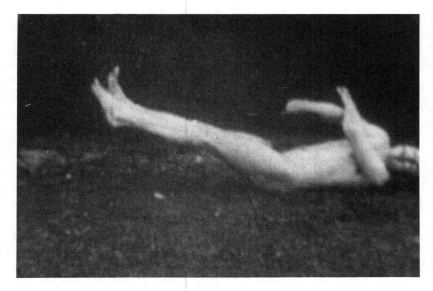

Figure 3.3. A case of status epilepticus, from the epilepsy biographs, Walter Greenough Chase (1905).

railway accidents. Hamilton shot motion picture films of many of these trauma victims and analyzed their movements in hopes of discerning the subtle physiological differences between cases of faked and real traumas.[29]

Although they did not go so far as to induce seizures mechanically or electrically in their patients, Spratling and Chase were also fascinated with distinctions between willed and involuntary, authentically pathological, movement. This interest is most apparent in their film of a case of status epilepticus, a potentially fatal form of epilepsy characterized by severe, relentless convulsions lasting sometimes for days. In his writings on the case, Chase explained that the ten-year-old boy who appears in the film suffered fifteen discrete seizures, all of them quite severe, culminating in a fifty-minute attack of status (figure 3.3). Camera wind and roll-film length were important factors in this study. Chase was able to capture on film only four of the fifty minutes of seizure. His account of the status epilepticus case exemplifies the range and extent of observational techniques used when film analysis alone was clearly not up to the task of total surveillance. In addition to frame enlargements, he provides charts, graphs, and written statistical analyses that give the time of day (to the second) of the seizure depicted; data on weight, height, and capabilities of hearing, sight, and speech; number and duration of past seizures; temperature, pulse, and respiration; and clinical signs (the state of the lungs, tongue, heart, skin, and eyes). Spratling too uses statistical methods to augment film analysis: he preceded his account of the

Chase films with a chart summarizing detailed data on seizures occurring in the colony population over the course of a year.[30]

In the face of this intensive management of seizure through multifarious surveillance techniques, status epilepticus presents a limit case, representing seizure without closure and loss of motor control potentially culminating in death. Indeed, the film is a metaphor for Spratling's own anxiety about neurology's inability to control epilepsy—an anxiety that is managed in an obsession with detail and a compulsion for repetition evident in the frame analysis or the film loop. Chase and Spratling documented not only every aspect of the seizure, but also its briefest moments and its smallest details. Chase computed the number of film frames in order to make it clear that he had accrued a vast quantity of information: he had thirty-seven thousand separate pictures, he boasted, thirty-two hundred of them documenting the rare case of status. He suggested that a flip book might be produced to facilitate repeated viewing of the images, and that the film projector magnifies "the biograph projection to life size" so that "the very action of the muscles may be studied." Clearly, for Chase, cinematography shared with more strictly clinical techniques like microscopy a tendency to detail and abstraction, facilitating obsessive close analysis. Spratling apparently shared this obsession. For him, the films were the fulfillment of many years' endeavor to "reproduce different types of seizures in the minutest detail" so that "even the saliva pouring from the mouth" would be visible.[31]

This obsession with detail suggests that Chase and Spratling thought that the cinematic motion study could help them determine epilepsy's etiology. But according to Spratling, etiologic investigation involved more than simply seeing and reading the image; it demanded an observer trained in isolating and decoding nearly imperceptible signs, signs that perhaps lay outside the province of the camera. In a passage that makes clear his awareness of a historical shift in the perception of epilepsy—and a shift in neurology's modes of perception—he suggested that the understanding of the condition has changed. The visual display of movement, he argues, is no longer epilepsy's most characteristic sign:

> We now know that the visible fit, in itself, is only a symptom of a condition frequently profound, and, what is worst of all, frequently most obscure.[32]

This passage suggests that subtle signs (involuntary movement during semi-consciousness, or moments of relative stasis) are particularly important indicators of pathological expression because they are coded at the margins of visibility. Hence they constitute data that may not yet be available to the neurologist trained to rely on visual observation. Given this view, it is difficult to understand Spratling's interest in visual analysis; moreover, it is difficult to understand why the most dramatic aspects of seizures were the main focus of Chase's films. This apparent disjuncture suggests that Chase and Spratling were caught up in a broader paradox of modern neurology: the need to calculate vectors of pathology that are not best characterized by visibility or fixed locale, through the discipline's traditional techniques of observation, recording, and classification.

As if to keep up with this new conception of pathology as mobile and elusive, Spratling used the biographs to identify those subtle signs missed in empirical observation. Unlike Charcot, who used serial images to compile general typologies of clinical signs, Spratling emphasized the need to study fleeting, minute details ("an unusual glitter of the eye," for example, or "a slight increase in the pulse rate") and the moments before convulsive movements rather than more obvious characteristics of the film images of fits.[33] He and Chase were interested less in the information offered in the moving image itself than in the difference between individual film frames and in the difference between normal and pathological movement that could be seen only when magnified by the projector. But even when used as a scientific instrument of measurement and analysis, Spratling implied, the biograph ultimately could not keep up with the specificity of modern forms of pathology. He suggested that it is finally neither cinematography nor neurology that is best equipped to produce new knowledge about epilepsy, but another scientific subspecialty altogether: chemical pathology. "I am convinced," he asserted,

> that the final elucidation of the great problem of the etiology of epilepsy lies in great part—I will go further and say in the greatest part—at the door of the chemical pathologist. I feel sure that we are bound to derive benefit more from the study of living matter—the blood, the urine, the stomach and intestinal contents, the sweat, etc.—in this question than from pathology only—than from any part of the body after it is dead.[34]

Spratling's argument is that the chemical pathologist, trained in techniques such as microscopy and chemical analysis, was far better equipped than the neurologist to read the interior processes of the body. The study of epilepsy thus shifted its locus beyond the study of dead tissue (autopsy) and beyond the cinematic record of the living surface (observation, motion analysis). "The study of living matter" for clues about epilepsy's etiology was now also the province of more specialized disciplines—those better equipped to work within the modern configuration of disease as a nonlocalized, mobile system. As Spratling put it, epilepsy's source eluded the modern neurological gaze:

> It is not a stable, fixed, definite, and, at this time, demonstrable cause that produces the convulsion, but something that comes and goes, that is most insidious—that is present to-day or this week, and absent to-morrow or the week after, and that often acts on an organism far below par.[35]

Of what use were the epilepsy biographs to Spratling, then, if they did not provide access to that which acts on the body "far below par"? A year before Chase produced the epilepsy biographs, Spratling made a strange assertion about the status of the seizure in the overall pathology, a statement that offers some insight into the regard of visible, external signs like the seizure. Rather than stating, as one might expect, that the seizure is a sign of pathology, he argued that it marks a moment of health in pathology's course through the body. The "purpose of the seizure is salutary," he explained; it is "a moment of release" that serves to counteract the "systemic poisoning" that takes place in the nervous system of the epileptic subject.[36] Whereas for Charcot, physical signs were external markers of interior pathology, Spratling saw these same external signs as *gaps* in pathology's signifying chain—as brief moments of health in the continuum of illness. Although Chase did not film patients between seizures, the scientists who worked in the colony's laboratory of chemical pathology emphasized the role of chemical change in the body at precisely these in-between times as opportune moments for investigation— opportune, that is, for the researcher equipped with analytic tools other than empirical observation.[37] The faculty of seeing and its instruments of visibility were no match for chemical action, the flow of the blood, or the electrical processes of the nervous system. It seems that at the time that Chase documented the most heightened visual manifestations of seizure, these were no longer regarded as the most etiologically telling aspects of the disease.

Spratling notes that the definition of epilepsy was changing in another important way: epilepsy was no longer a unified disease, but a disorder without a singular etiology. Like Charcot's hysteria, Spratling's epilepsy defied neurological investigation and classification. In a talk delivered before a presentation of the epilepsy biographs to the Philadelphia College of Physicians, Spratling states that despite intensive analysis of the sort represented in Chase's biographs, epilepsy simply could not be classified etiologically, but had to be classified by its symptomatology. In fact, he explained, epilepsy is a multifarious entity: "The day has gone by when we can speak of epilepsy. We must speak of the epilepsies."[38]

"The epilepsies" as Spratling describes them are organized chiefly around gender poles: there are male epilepsies and there are female epilepsies. So far, I have focused on the eighteen biographs of male epileptics. However, Chase also produced three short films of women diagnosed as "hysteroepileptics." Though they differ stylistically from the films of men, they are included in Chase's compilation reel and discussed in his essays. Leslie Camhi emphasizes that "the cadaverizing gaze was for nineteenth-century medicine the special prerogative of feminine sexuality." There is, she continues, "a subtle encoding of feminized bodies in the pure materiality of epileptic movement and uncontrolled musculature" of both male and female epileptics.[39] While it is certainly true that the men herded together and paraded nude before the camera were subject to sadistic and voyeuristic modes of spectatorship, it is the more subtle images of women epileptics that seem to embody Spratling's concept of the epilepsies. I now consider the films of women epileptics in order to demonstrate that, more than the biographs of men, these images of women epileptics embodied both a modern understanding of epilepsy as a condition characterized in terms of duration (as defined by Spratling) and neurology's own anxieties about visual observation, recording, and analysis. Though quite sedate compared to the films of the men, Chase's biographs of women patients come closest to demonstrating Spratling's theory of epilepsy as an elusive, unstable, mobile, and insidious disease; they function in part as metaphorical expressions of the state of knowledge in the field of neurology.

Spratling associated epilepsy in men with social factors: "If a man escapes syphilis, alcoholism, and injury to the brain, he is not likely to have epilepsy." He viewed alcohol, illness, or brain injury as inductive forces that, like the neurologist's electrical or mechanical stimulation, cause seizure. However, he also cited hereditary predisposition as a factor. For example, he attributed the case of status epilepticus described above to parental abuse but then noted that "the hereditary influence was bad, parents having been alcoholic and very nervous."[40] It appears that the "great degenerescence system" was still functioning in Spratling's scheme.

If male epileptics were regarded as social degenerates, the condition of epilepsy in women was viewed as both degenerate and innate. Spratling attributed epilepsy in women not to social or organic causes but to biological factors and genetic inheritance:

> More epilepsies occur in the 12th to 15th year than in any other period. This is especially true in women. At the Craig Colony we have performed much abdominal surgery in cases in which the seizures grouped themselves about the menstrual period. We have had some excellent results. We look for a neurotic ancestry in such cases.[41]

Chase's definition of epilepsy in women designated "hysteroepileptics" clearly draws on Charcot's construction of hysteria as an innate condition resulting from a degenerate hereditary disposition, and reinforces the nineteenth-century pathologizing of non-Western peoples and all women that Stepan describes. The term is applied not only to women patients, but also to one man—a patient who is identified as black. The symptoms of the one black man described in Spratling's text (but not imaged in Chase's films) are described, like those of the women, in terms that render him all but incurable. Although white male epileptics are designated degenerate, their condition is not considered innate and is even regarded as potentially self-correcting (as I will show in a moment). However, the hysteroepilepsy purportedly borne by the women and the black man is regarded as innate, degenerate, and incurable—manageable only through the intervention of surgery.

The biographs of women designated hysteroepileptics are stylistically closer to the Salpêtrière photographs than to Chase's biographs of men. In the three films of women, Chase's subjects appear, like Charcot's hysterics, in their everyday clothing and are shot in medium close-up so that we can see their expressions in detail. Though they stand facing the camera, they avert their eyes from its line of sight. But there is at least one important difference between these films and the Salpêtrière iconographies: We see in the biographs neither the stylized poses depicted in the iconographies of women hysterics nor the extreme contortions of seizure shown in the biographs of epileptic men. Rather, we see athetosis—that is, slow, continual, and involuntary writhing, particularly of the hands and arms. In Spratling's view, these are the subtle signs that are apparent only to the trained observer, the signs that characterize that multifarious modern disorder, the epilepsies.

Linda Williams's analysis of Eadweard Muybridge's motion studies of human physiology offers a useful perspective on the epilepsy biographs. She suggests that in Muybridge's serial photographs women's bodies are most often invested with an iconographic or diegetic surplus of meaning. The female body is provided with gendered garb (dresses, hats), domestic props (brooms, buckets), and a domestic or sexualized narrative context (sweeping, bathing). In contrast, the men are most often photographed (as in Chase's films) unclothed or nearly nude, performing mechanical actions without the detailed mise-en-scène and narrative causality we see in the images of women—except in cases where masculine scenarios (sports and battle scenes, for example) are staged ostensibly to elicit particular muscular and kinetic activity. Adhering to the pictorial codes of science (neutral backdrop, nude bodies, no props other than those used to induce or measure the movement studied), the images of men are coded to read as textbook cases of anatomy and physiology. By contrast, the women, surrounded by gender-specific props, accoutrements, and narratives, are marked "as more embedded within a socially prescribed system of objects and gestures."[42]

The women in the epilepsy biographs are also made to bear an iconographic surplus of meaning. They are framed and clothed in a style consistent with the photographic iconography of hysteria. Their movements, restrained and graceful when compared with the frenetic movements we see in the films of the men, are encoded as both more feminine and more akin to voluntary, signifying movements (figures 3.4 and 3.5). These images are strikingly similar to some of the motion studies of hysteria published in France during this period. For example, in a series of photographs that illustrate Fulgence Raymond and Pierre Janet's *Névroses et idées fixes*, we see a mock dance in a case of chorea in which the woman faces the camera frontally and appears to exhibit a structured performance for the camera (figure 3.6).[43]

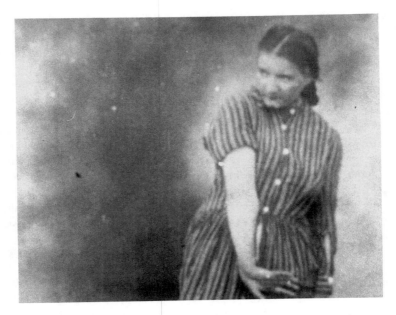

Figure 3.4. Frame from the epilepsy biographs, Walter Greenough Chase (1905).

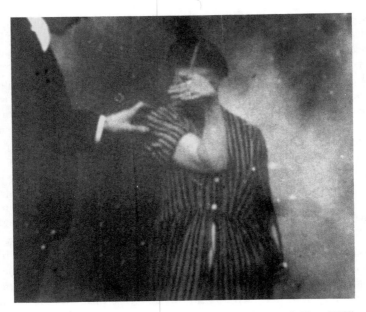

Figure 3.5. Frame from the epilepsy biographs, Walter Greenough Chase (1905).

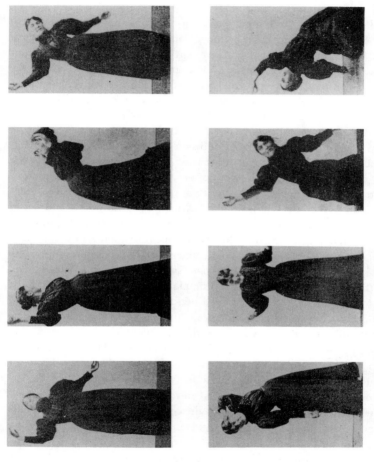

Figure 3.6. A mock dance in a case of chorea. From Fulgence Raymond and Pierre Janet, *Névroses et idée fixes* (Paris: Félix Alcan, 1898).

Clearly the films of women are made to bear a closer resemblance to "normal" performances of movement. Yet it is the men's seizures, and not the women's, that are imbued with stronger narrative causality and closure. Spratling, as we have seen, argued that the seizure serves the purpose of cleansing the system of poisons generated by external stimulus (alcohol, injury, abuse). This idea of cleansing suggests a narrative progression that is absent in the biographs of women. The men's seizures have a clear beginning (we see them in the unconscious state, out of control) and a conclusion (at the end of many takes, the men regain self-control—they rise or appear to address offscreen personnel). Although the men initially appear more out of control, we are told that they are in fact experiencing a healthy, cathartic release from pathology. We are not, however, given the chance to see the women return to self-determined action and social interchange, even for a moment. Though the medium close-up gives us a clearer view of their facial expressions in seizure and provides a stronger sense of the patient's individuality and subjectivity, there is no point at which the women appear to note the presence of camera or audience, no sign of an imminent return to cognizant social engagement. Apparently the seizures of hysteroepilepsy are not healthy or do not purge the body of poisons, like the seizures of the men.

There is another important difference in the presentation of male and female seizures. While the gestures of the men are quite erratic and hence potentially difficult to codify, the women's athetotic movements appear relatively ordered and systematic. They almost seem to approximate a kind of gestural language. The films of women epileptics compare interestingly with a 1904 Edison Company film, *Deaf-Mute Girl Reciting the Star-Spangled Banner*. In this film, a woman clothed in a simple country dress (not unlike those worn by the colony women) is filmed performing elaborate hand and arm movements, also against a cloth backdrop (an oversized American flag). The title of the film lets the viewer know that the woman is in fact using her body to sing—or, rather, to sign—the national anthem. The gestures of the woman are meaningful even to those not versed in sign language. They signify at the very least a visual substitute for vocal performance; as such, the performance is a metaphor for the silent cinema, itself a "deaf-mute" signifying system that relies almost wholly on the construction of somatic signs, the honing of physiology to a kind of visual enunciation in the absence of sound technology.

The Biograph Company film seems to suggest that film itself may function prosthetically to extend the incomplete body of the sensorily impaired spectator. In 1891, near the end of his ten-year assistantship to Marey, Georges Demenÿ had already produced a series of chronophotographic images meant to perform precisely this function for the deaf. In an extreme close-up of his own mouth, Demenÿ silently mouthed the phrase "Je vous aime." This series of frames was projected, by means of a phenakistoscope, to a hearing-impaired audience, who successfully read Demenÿ's lips.[44] In this instance, the motion picture functioned as a prosthetic aid to audition. Demenÿ's project suggests that the visual representation of voice bore more than a symbolic or metaphorical meaning. This greater meaning is also evident in the early development of cinema sound technology. In 1885, Alexander Graham Bell patented a device for the deaf through which manometric flames from a gas jet regulated by sound waves generated by voice could be photographically recorded and read. This technique would be incorporated in the cinema's earliest optical soundtracks, which also relied on the reproduction of graphically recorded patterns.

Chase, again working with Biograph Company equipment, drew on this association of the cinema image and sound in another film project. Working with doctors at the Massachusetts Home for the Feeble-Minded, he filmed a group he described as "rhythmic idiots, each with his individual motion and keeping time to music."[45] The relatively recent availability of regulated filming and projection rate established a technological standard of rhythm in the film image, setting off the marked arrhythmia of the patients filmed. If the arrhythmic movements of the patients emphasize the absence of an audible musical pattern, and hence the absence of a standard against which to verify the arrhythmia of movements, the visual rhythm of projection stands in for such a standard. As in the Edison film, the motion study is used to depict an uncomfortable state between motor incoordination and signification. Signifying absence of regulation in the presence of "pure" mechanical movement, the body filmed becomes an explicit figure for the failure of the mechanical to bear directed meaning in the aural register. The *Deaf-Mute Girl Reciting the Star-Spangled Banner*, the woman and the film alike, is ultimately contained within signification through regulated movement even in the presence of sensory impairment (on the part of technology and subject) at the level of speech and sound; however, the absence signified in the Chase films by the apparent lapse between neural and motor process, as well as between image and its portrayal of sound, exerts a threat of a living death. The possibility of perceiving the cinema as a machine through which to regulate or extend life is circumvented by these lapses.

The women in the epilepsy biographs similarly enunciate through a gestural performance; however, their somatic gestures remain at the margins of signification. Their involuntary movements are to a great degree arbitrary in meaning. However, as in the Edison film, these gestures also enunciate the state of visuality in the field. Like the iconographic gestures of the "singing"/signing woman, the movements of the epileptic women signify a methodological lack. Just as the signing woman cannot bring voice to the silent cinema, so the gesticulating woman cannot make the moving image express the nature and etiology of her condition for her audience of neurologists and physicians.

The Neurological Cinematographic Atlas

A little more than a decade after Chase produced his epilepsy biographs, the U.S. neurophysiologist Frederick Tilney developed a cinematic technique for analyzing movement disorders. He called his method bradykinetic analysis (*brady* means "slow"). Following Chase's precedent, Tilney used slow-speed projection to analyze what he called his "cinematographs." Tilney's studies allow us to look more closely at neurology's attempt to construct an etiology of organic illness with the help of the moving image. He began his studies in 1918, the first year of a major six-year epidemic in the United States of lethargic encephalitis (sleeping sickness), a viral disease that caused thousands of deaths throughout the world around the time of the First World War. As already noted, lethargic encephalitis virtually disappeared from clinical studies for decades during this century, not for lack of patients, but because it "could not be accommodated in the conventional frameworks" of neurological knowledge.[46] And as suggested earlier, lethargic encephalitis confounded neurological analysis in part because it involved organic factors during a period when psychological causation was a favored diagnosis. Encephalitis caused severe, and in many cases irreversible, damage to the brain and spinal cord. The nature of neurological damage due to encephalitis was difficult to discern because in many cases symptoms appeared years after the illness. As with Tourette syndrome, postencephalitic symptoms were hard to pin down because, in many cases, neurologists could not distinguish them from those of disorders understood to be psychogenic in origin, and hence not in the province of neurology, but belonging to the realm of psychiatry or psychoanalysis.[47] Responding to the proliferation of nervous and mental diseases between the wars, neurologists attempted to maintain order by encoding perceived distinctions among organic, genetic, and psychogenic diseases. Tilney used bradykinetic analysis throughout the six-year epidemic to discern subtleties of movement that might help him make such distinctions.

In 1944, two Columbia University neurophysiologists, S. Philip Goodhart and Benjamin Harris Balser, published the *Neurological Cinematographic Atlas* to accompany a series of films, including Tilney's early experiments in bradykinetic analysis. They wanted to document what had been learned about nervous diseases in the years between the wars—years marked by the prevalence of encephalitis and the rise in popularity of psychoanalysis.[48] The writings and film series of Goodhart and Balser provide one of the clearest examples of the use of the physiological film motion study during this period and through the Second World War. But, more importantly, they make absolutely clear the limitations of diagnosis through organic signs and visual images. Whereas Chase and Spratling expressed some hope in learning something new about the physiological nature of nervous pathology through their motion studies, Goodhart and Balser's films exhibit a visceral anxiety around the neurologist's ability to know the nervous system, their privileged domain. This anxiety centers on the epistemological status of visuality, the distinction between organic and psychogenic disorders, and the ability to establish a clear etiologic narrative for elusive organic diseases like encephalitis.

A 1944 film included in the atlas, *Dystonia Musculorum Deformans*, compiles footage shot by Tilney for bradykinetic analysis between 1929 and 1935 and footage of the same patient shot by Goodhart and Balser years later. Intertitles explain that the woman presented in the film was initially diagnosed as suffering from a disorder of psychogenic origins but that while using bradykinetic analysis to analyze her movements, Tilney saw subtle, nearly imperceptible wavelike movements rippling through the muscles of the thigh. These "vermicular" (wormlike) movements, intertitles explain, are typical of a particular postencephalitic disease: dystonia musculorum deformans (DMD), or torsion dystonia. The film thus demonstrated to Tilney and his colleagues the claim made by Spratling, Chase, and other neurologists that the motion study could uniquely provide key visual evidence in the construction of an etiology.

DMD is marked by involuntary contortions of the trunk and extremities—movements described in the medical literature as grotesque. A point not noted in the film is that the disease is also described in the medical literature as a rare genetic illness occurring in a recessive form principally among Jews.[49] It is significant that a disease held to be genetically recessive among Jews happens to be the focus of a neurological film motion study produced in the United States in 1944, during the period of Nazi medical practice in Germany. According to the medical film historian Adolph Nichtenhauser, neuropsychiatry was the medical specialty in which film production developed most extensively in Germany after World War I.[50] German neurological films of this period are evidence of the continued prevalence of the empiricism-visuality conjuncture and the racist system of degenerescence in twentieth-century science. Many of these films were produced to serve as evidence of racial degeneracy in epilepsy and other disorders and to support arguments for methods such as enforced sterilization before euthanasia committees and nonmedical audiences. Neuropsychiatry was a critical field in the attempt to legitimate Nazi eugenics.[51]

Goodhart and Balser's decision to focus on a disease held to be genetically recessive among Jews cannot be seen apart from this broader disciplinary context. This point is reinforced by the fact that their colleague, Ernst Herz, had studied with Karl Kleist, a major figure in German neurology who produced numerous motion studies of mental diseases. After emigrating to the United States in the 1930s, Herz produced a series of ten silent teaching films, accompanied in 1946 by a book, *Motor Disorders in Nervous Diseases*.

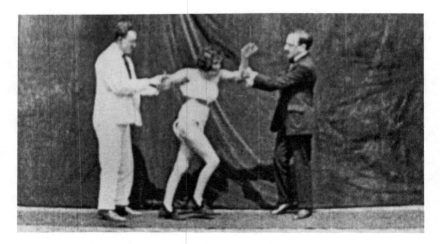

Figure 3.7. Frame from *Dystonia Musculorum Deformans* (1944).

This series is quite similar to the studies of epilepsy, encephalitis, and other diseases filmed by Kleist and his colleagues between 1924 and the early 1940s. This is not to say that Herz, his partner Tracy Putnam, or Goodhart and Balser were implicated in Nazi medical agendas; rather, U.S. neurology at midcentury also continued to participate in the construction of racist and sexist visual typologies—a project that extended across Western science. Indeed, frame enlargements from films produced at the Kleist Clinic appear in *Motor Disorders in Nervous Diseases* with the disclaimer that the German images are "the property of the world of biological science"—as if one could transcend the methods and circumstances of their production.

But the adoption of the images and techniques of German neurology into U.S. practice was not wholesale. Herz and his colleagues also relied on psychoanalysis to support their case studies. This peculiar joining of psychoanalysis and empirical neurology suggests that the advance of psychoanalysis over biologism described by Rose was uneven at best. The revolutionary new science certainly did not make itself wholly incommensurate with neurology. Goodhart and Balser's atlas of nervous diseases is evidence of the interface, perhaps even the necessary interdependency, between neurology and psychoanalysis at a time during which the latter discipline had gained authority. In the following analysis of two of the films in the neurological atlas I foreground the problems that arose with Goodhart and Balser's insistence on psychogenic causality and its structuring paternal law in the search for an etiology of organic pathology.

Goodhart and Balser's filmic record of DMD begins with a demonstration of Tilney's diagnostically successful use of bradykinetic analysis. We see the original footage of the woman at actual speed, in which irregular leg move-

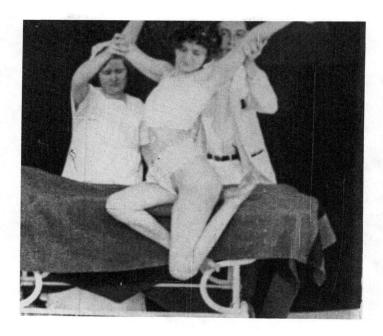

Figure 3.8. Frame from *Dystonia Musculorum Deformans* (1944).

ment is evident (figure 3.7). Then we see the same footage slowed down to reveal that the irregular movement comprises a rippling or wavelike formation invisible at standard projection rate. The film then turns from analytical footage to case documentation, from which it soon becomes apparent that prognosis, treatment, and even etiology were beyond Tilney's reach. We see that the woman's condition progressively worsened, her movements becoming more and more irregular. Unable to still the degenerative process, the neurologists responded with a most bizarre treatment. In an attempt to suppress her symptomatic movements, they weighed down their patient's legs with heavy plaster casts. Tilney's idea was to train the body to function without its tremor, and to force it to move without the contortions characteristic of the disease—physical restraint as physical therapy.

Goodhart and Balser continued to film this woman throughout the early 1940s as her movement disorder regressed toward complete loss of motor control. However, their documentation of movement differs radically from the films of Tilney a decade earlier. Just as Tilney attempted to cure the ailment by forcing the symptomatic movement to cease, Goodhart and Balser also attempted to freeze pathological movement. They physically pin down the woman's body, fixing her in a series of erotic poses meant to signify typical configurations of pathology (figure 3.8). In groups of two and three, the medical staff struggles to arrange this woman's disorderly body, anxious to

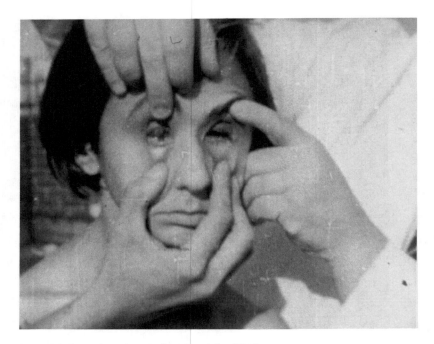

Figure 3.9. Frame from *Acute Epidemic Encephalitis* (1944).

freeze for the motion picture camera a fixed iconic register of uncontrolled movement. But these iconic poses, making up a compendium of signs of pathology, provide neither knowledge nor cure. For the neurologists, the return to the static icon covers over the inevitable fact of their own loss of control over movement and signification, and the shortcomings of their own techniques and instruments.

In *Acute Epidemic Encephalitis*, another entry in Goodhart and Balser's atlas of nervous diseases, an emaciated young woman with empty eye cavities and a toothless mouth and wearing only a diaperlike garment is paraded before the camera by a male attendant. Next we see two close-ups of the woman, one in which her mouth is pried open to reveal the absence of her teeth, and another in which her eye sockets are forced open by the hands of the attendant to reveal empty cavities (figure 3.9). The case history reported in the intertitles explains that the woman featured in this film, who had suffered encephalitis many years ago, had suddenly and inexplicably performed the horrendous acts of extracting her teeth and eyes with her own hands. In the course of the film, we are also shown a close up of the two extracted eyeballs, their optic nerves intact, displayed lying side by side on a dark surface (figure 3.10). I quote from the case history written by Goodhart and his colleague Nathan Savitsky:

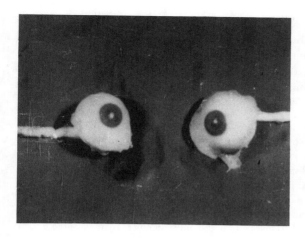

Figure 3.10. Frame from *Acute Epidemic Encephalitis* (1944).

[Some time during her early teen years, the patient] was admitted to Morisania Hospital because of some swelling and redness of the right eye. The mother noticed that she had been rubbing that eye during the day and there was some swelling and bulging. Her temperature was 100F.; pulse, 100; respirations, 22. She was examined by one of the house physicians, put to bed, her eye washed with boric acid and an ice-bag was applied. She was quiet and apparently slept until 3:20 AM, July 31. The nurse in charge of the ward states as follows: "I was notified by an attendant that this patient's eye had fallen out. I immediately went to the patient and found that she was holding her right eye in her hand and on questioning her she said that it had spontaneously fallen out while she was sleeping. She answered all my questions unhesitatingly and appeared intelligent. She did not complain of any pain or discomfort. Her actions were quite normal except for her seeming indifference toward the incident.[52]

This description is immediately followed by an analysis that breaks with neurological tradition by introducing material from two other areas: psychoanalysis and mythology. "Self-injury by avulsion of one's eyes is rare," the authors write, "though known to legend in the Oedipus story, and [in the story of] the self-mutilation of the patron saint of eye diseases, Santa Lucia."[53] It is highly significant that Goodhart and Savitsky select two accounts that foreground the correspondence of sexuality and vision (precisely the conjuncture that concerns Rose in her reading of Freud and Charcot). The mythological self-avulsion of the eyes by Oedipus is a familiar referent in discussions of male sexuality, and I shall consider it at greater length in a moment. But the comparison of this case to the Santa Lucia legend is most salient. While in one rendition of the story Lucia's eyes are torn out by her judges in punishment for her refusal of a suitor, in another Lucia tears out her own eyes to present them to a suitor she disliked who had admired them.[54] Which interpretation might the authors have favored in their comparison? This question is a crucial one; on its answer rides the difference between a reading of the event as a case of self-punishment or as an act of willful defiance. But Goodhart, Balser, and Savitsky leave us hanging, choosing instead to pursue the mythology of psychoanalysis to interpret their case.

In the publication that serves as a companion to the film, Balser and Goodhart emphasize that this woman's actions were in fact quite normal in almost all respects:

> Mentally she was cooperative in ward routine although displaying some irritability and mental instability. There were no spontaneous productions and her stream of thought was normal; she had no delusions or hallucinations and no bizarre ideas. Her affective reactions were apparently adequate and there was no dissociation of affect. She showed a real sense of humor and was much interested in what was going on. . . . Her reaction to discussion of her self-mutilation would be that of momentary depression and she avoided any reference to the episodes. She invariably stated that she did not remember anything of the period during which her eyes, as she expressed it, "popped out."[55]

Goodhart and Balser repeatedly cite examples of this woman's docility and compliance as indications of her health. Apparently her belief that her eyes had just "popped out" was not considered a delusion or a "bizarre idea" but a demonstration of her mental stability. Indeed, even her apparently easy acceptance of her loss of vision is presented as a sign of her stability and normalcy. She was an "apt pupil," we are told, who quickly learned to read through the Braille system shortly after the loss of her eyes.[56]

In their analysis of the case, Goodhart and Savitsky feminize the Oedipus myth to construct an etiology of this strange case of postacute encephalitis. They refer to Karl Abraham's 1920–22 "Manifestations of the Female Castration Complex." Regarding women's eyes, Abraham had the following to say:

> Some neurotic women get a marked congestion of the eyes with every sexual excitation. In a certain measure this congestion is a normal and common phenomenon accompanying sexual excitation. However, in those women of whom we are speaking the condition is not simply a quantitative increase of the phenomenon for a short period, but a redness of the sclerotics accompanied by a burning sensation, while swelling persists for several days after each sexual excitation. In such cases we are justified in speaking of a *conjunctivitis neurotica*.[57]

Though they make no reference to this relevant passage in their mention of the castration complex, Goodhart and Savitsky could not have overlooked it in their selection of this text as a reference in the case history. Their adoption of a psychoanalytic paradigm in itself is perplexing. It suggests a belief that a psychogenic model may function within neurology as a literal historical instance, a parallel case history. Such an understanding of case history is strikingly out of place, especially in the treatment of a case where organic causation has been so carefully documented. The case history indicates that it was not sexual excitation that had caused the "marked congestion of the eyes" in the woman, but encephalitis. One would think that the two could not be so easily confused. Goodhart writes that this woman suffered repeated ocular disturbances throughout her life after bouts of illness, and exhibited other severe motor disturbances characteristic of postencephalitis. What was diagnosed as "weakness of the eyes" following a severe illness was followed by a total lack of accommodation in one eye and sluggishness in the other. The case history presents clear evidence of organic impairment of sight as an important component of this woman's eventual self-enucleation. Why, then, the shift in focus to the mythological, and to Abraham's highly sexualized account of "conjunctivitis neurotica," a female neurosis of the eyes brought on by sexual excitation? Even if the authors intend Abraham's account to function metaphorically, the implication would stand that, regardless of its origins, self-enucleation cannot be read outside the cultural convergence of vision, sexuality, and knowledge. At the base of Goodhart and Savitsky's case history is the idea that, regardless of the organic factors involved, self-enucleation is an act of profound epistemological significance, an instance of the most extreme self-denial of sexual pleasure and knowledge. There is no implication of any awareness that, for this sufferer of encephalitis, the eyes might have been the site of another order of experience—for example, unbearable physical pain.

I offer instead an alternative reading of this text. We are told that this patient experienced an analgesic absenting of pain following her extraction of teeth and eyes. According to her own account, the removal of her eyes was what eased her symptoms. This woman's act implies that the faculty of sight is not worth the ocular pain she suffered. The fact that she would opt to forgo sight is repulsive to Goodhart and Savitsky precisely because it signifies to them an unthinkable state of existence: to lack the knowledge and pleasure afforded by the eye. The woman they filmed was a visceral embodiment of this unthinkable condition. For the male viewer deeply invested in visual knowledge, the empty, scarred eye cavities marking the face of this woman are a particularly charged signifier of castration. Like the male child in Freud's account of the origins of castration anxiety, the neurologist must manage this symbolic sight of castration by retrospectively constructing narratives that temper and recast the brutal knowledge it conveys. Perhaps it is in fact the neurologist who experiences a case of conjunctivitis neurotica: traumatized as he is by a sight worse than castration itself, he must manage his anxieties about visuality and knowledge by disavowing the horrendous scene.

I return for a moment to the 1905 epilepsy biographs. At the end of one of Chase's studies, the young man being filmed regains consciousness and looks and gestures toward the camera. The shot abruptly ends, eliding from the record the subject's attempt to return, comprehendingly, the neurologist's look. I would not go so far as to say that this moment documents an instance of resistance to the medicalized surveillance to which this patient is subjected. But the neurologist's rejection of the patient's comprehending gaze represented in this cut can be interpreted in retrospect as a moment of professional unease over this look back at the camera. The neurological filmmaker is made uncomfortable by the comprehending look of the patient, not because her look challenges the authority of his gaze, but because it reminds him of his own inability to discipline the bodies of his charges, to make them perform their illnesses on cue and involuntarily. Goodhart and Savitsky's film marks a significant moment in the history of the neurological gaze. If at the turn of the century the neurologist was unable to render the body docile and compliant, by midcentury the neurologist is unable to make his own body perform its duties within the apparatus of the scientific gaze. The self-enucleated woman mirrors the state of the postwar neurologist. He is himself a figure stripped of his ability to control and direct the operations of the disciplinary gaze. By midcentury, the cinema camera, with its singular viewpoint and its supervisory camera operator behind the lens, is no longer an adequate instrument for the task of managing organic illness.

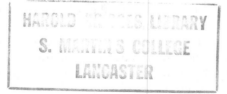

CHAPTER 4

A Microphysics of the Body: Microscopy and the Cinema

WHAT CAN YOU TELL about a man without seeing him, say, from an examination of the photo?" asked Robert Lincoln Watkins, a New York physician, in a publication of 1902. The photo in question is not a conventional portrait but a photomicrograph—an image shot through the lens of the microscope. "I cannot tell . . . what he looks like in the face any more than the ancients could judge Socrates by his looks," Watkins explained, "but I think there is some disintegration taking place in the man." He goes on to make a detailed diagnosis of the man's condition based on the appearance of the blood cells in the image. What does it mean that, for this doctor, the site of diagnosis has shifted from body surface to the blood cells? Like Spratling, Watkins believed that the site where the researcher can most effectively uncover insidious signs of pathology is neither the body surface nor its interior organs and structures but a non-site-specific fluid: "In the blood lies more disease as well as more premonitory symptoms of disease than can be found in any other part of the body," he asserted. "He is the greatest discoverer who finds the pre-symptom or the symptom of the symptom," those "slight and unconscious departures from a normality."[1]

Though Watkins was not a well-known or influential physician, his account functions as a useful caricature of the physiological foray into the body during this period. Hooking up his patients to a "micromotoscope," an instrument of his design that combined microscope and movie camera, he observed their blood in living action, describing with great exuberance its appearance as it flowed from vein to specimen plate, where its microscopic movement was recorded by the movie camera.[2] Like Chase, Watkins wrote of splicing his film into a loop that, under projection, would make the blood appear to flow as if it were still alive. He was apparently unaware that the movement he observed was not the activity of living blood at all but the drift of dead blood cells through the inert solution that coated the glass slide. What is most remarkable, however, is not this mistaking of death for life, but Watkins's drive quite literally to draw an imperceptible living process out of the body and expect it to perform its own pathology, splayed out flat on the microscope's aptly named stage. If Watkins saw disintegration taking place in the man whose photomicrograph he viewed, this disintegration was engendered by the microscope itself, through its techniques of bodily fragmentation and abstraction.

It is not surprising that the Craig Colony's researchers regarded the living blood as the key distinguishing factor in the identification of their elusive and multifarious object, the epilepsies. The epileptic and the hysteroepileptic, colony pathologists argued, could be told apart only by "differences in the condition of the blood."[3] This focus on the blood, a fluid and unstable vehicle for the passage of matter throughout the body, is a distinctly physiological way of conceiving of the body. But the blood is also a broader metaphor for the object of medical perception. No longer concerned with the body as such, medicine is interested in isolating life—in regulating and extending it, and in gaining control over death in the process. The observed body comes to be viewed as a vehicle, a site of living processes. Accordingly, the sensory body of the medical observer and its perceptual apparatus must accommodate its object, itself becoming more properly physiological. Sight must become more like the blood: fluid, pervasive, and unfixed from a locale. The researcher's sense of sight is thus subject to all manner of technological augmentation, displacement, and verification; its authority is dispersed across instruments like the kymograph, the cinematograph, and the microscope. Perception becomes unhinged from the sensory body and is enacted across an increasingly complex battery of institutional techniques and instruments.

This chapter is about physiology's animated quest to chart the body's imperceptible nonsites (blood flow, minute tissue growth, nerve action) and its deployment of perceptual instruments celebrated for their ability to vivify the body: the microscope and cinematography. I consider the work of scientists who used the microscope and the motion picture camera together to capture subtle events taking place, to use Spratling's phrase, "far below par," outside the range of visibility. In the laboratory practices I consider here, the microscopic motion picture is more than a representation of imperceptible living processes, and more than a scientific metaphor of life. It is a mechanism through which science reorganized its conception of the living body, ultimately rendering the physical body a more viewer-friendly site—but a site whose appearance was radically reordered to reflect the body's new status as a mobile, living system. As a means of monitoring and regulating processes such as the growth of tissue and vascular structure at their earliest stages and in their minutest detail, the cinemicroscopic apparatus is implicated in the growth of fields like microbiology and bioengineering during this century—fields that engage in the technological analysis and manufacture of new kinds of bodies and new forms of life.

In the following pages I attempt to describe the particular configuration of the medical gaze in early- to mid-twentieth-century microscopic cinematography, a configuration that existed simultaneously with the neurological gaze and its more conventionally pictorial and narrative forms. I try to show that the classificatory systems that informed normative models of health in terms of sexuality, gender, and cultural identity during this period were as central to cinematic microscopic images as they were to the more conventional pictorial images of neurological patients considered in the previous chapter. Whereas the motion picture of the eyeless, toothless body of the woman considered at the close of the previous chapter unquestionably repels and shocks, the image of a sliced, stained, and magnified fragment of body tissue is more likely to elicit viewer responses ranging from lack of interest to mild curiosity, or even aesthetic appreciation. In fields such as chemical pathology and hematology, the body is segmented, drained, sliced, and otherwise fragmented, the microscope rendering its minute fragments largely unidentifiable except to the specialized viewer. Placing a specimen on the instrument's stage and closing one eye to peer through the viewfinder, the microscopist sees the body in a manner that effectively distances the observer from the subjective experience of the body imaged. Excised from the body, stained, blown up, resolved, pierced by a penetrating light, and perceived by a single squinting eye, the microscopic specimen is apparently stripped of its corporeality, its function, and its history even as it serves as a final proof of the health, pathology, or sexuality of the subject whose body it represents. The purpose of this chapter, then, is to trace this dissolution of the corporeal body and its subject in the history of the microscopic image. What I offer is essentially a microhistory of a technical culture—an account that zeroes in on the minutiae of this particular subspecialty of medical science. In looking to the specific, it is my intention to uncover those places where the microscopic gaze has most tidily excised the matter of its own role as an instrument of institutional surveillance and power. Microscopy closes one eye to its object, offering up a modernist text that is stripped of historical as much as spatial depth. Twentieth-century microscopic imaging provides examples of medical visual culture at its slickest and its most aesthetically polished; the following is an attempt to rough up the smooth modernist surface of the microscopic image in order to uncover a history encoded in the interstices of this complexly layered field.

It is commonly held that microscopy prosthetically augments the range of the scientific observer's vision, allowing the perception of deep, minute, mobile, and generally imperceptible structures and entities. This evolutionary narrative of technology as visual aid does not begin with modernity, nor even with the Enlightenment. Pick up almost any history of microbiology and you will find a narrative that begins with Anton van Leeuwenhoek and his jubilant seventeenth-century sightings of "animalcules" swimming under the single lens of his magnifying instrument.[4] These histories invite an analysis of the genealogy of masculine fascination with the exaggerated image of minuscule bodily organisms (not surprisingly, sperm was a popular performer on the early microscopic stage); however, more pressing still is the need to analyze the microscopist's perpetual drive to correct, dissect, and retool the apparatus—the living organisms they viewed, and the instruments and bodies that facilitated that vision. The magnified image that delighted the technical eye was subjected to a relay of corrective gazes embedded in the instrument. As Jonathan Crary has shown, by the nineteenth century technical observation had already moved beyond the camera–obscura model of embodied vision, centralized gaze, and singular viewpoint to embrace techniques that dispersed power across a range of methods, instruments, and viewpoints.[5] Although by the nineteenth century microscopy still involved a singular monocular observer, that observer's perception was nevertheless continually corrected and calibrated by the apparatus just as the observer supervised and calibrated the bodies whose fragments were observed.

The Microscopic Apparatus

Technical literature on microscopy is quick to point out that it was the ability to resolve the magnified image, and not the sight of invisible entities in itself, that truly excited scientists.[6] Magnification is measured by the ratio of image size to specimen size. With their simple lenses, early microscopists were able to get enlarged views of tiny organisms. But they could not be sure that the blurry images they saw corresponded accurately to the invisible entity positioned under the lens. The representational microscopic image differs from the representational painting or photograph in that its accuracy cannot be confirmed against the human eye's view of its object.

Without detail and resolution, its accuracy unable to be judged against a perceived real, the view of the invisible provided by the early single-lens microscope was a source of epistemological instability and anxiety. The development of the compound microscope (after 1600) was regarded as a critical breakthrough for scientific microscopy because it introduced a means of resolving and correcting the magnified image. In the compound microscope, a second lens is positioned behind the magnifying lens. By adjusting its position, the microscopist could sharpen the view and increase its detail. The implantation of this second, analyzing lens signaled a shift in the culture of microscopy. The thrill of the spectacle of life was replaced by the intellectual stimulation of close inspection. Magnifying lens and observer's eye both became part of a new compound apparatus. But if the single lens of the simple microscope prosthetically augmented the eye of the observer by extending its range of vision, it also made it impossible to ignore the observer's dependency on technology. The compound lens system took this subjection of the observer's eye a step further, calibrating and correcting its subjective perception.

The compound microscope functions in much the same way as the nineteenth-century astronomical chronograph described at length by Shaffer (discussed in chapter 2), an instrument that kept in line the ostensibly flawed subjective perceptions of the human observer, relegating the observer's eye to the margins in the management of an otherwise optically inaccessible realm. Invested with the agency previously afforded the human eye, the astronomical chronograph and the microscope both can be regarded as arbiters of knowledge of inaccessible space, from the infinite to the infinitesimal. But if the magnifying lens stood firmly and irrefutably between the observer and the microscopic, the compound lens effectively confused the relation between observer and instrument by moving the arbitration of the image inside the instrument itself. It would no longer be a singular instrument that stands between observer and observed, but a heterogeneous apparatus through which the object-image is successively rendered and restructured, even before it is subject to the scrutiny of the microscopist's eye. Though not part of the instrument per se, the monocular viewing subject's perceptions would be overdetermined within the self-regulating gaze of the institutional apparatus.

Though it was introduced as a corrective to the problems of magnification, the resolving lens generated as many anxieties as it dispelled. The historian of microscopy G. L'E. Turner points out that the earliest compound microscopes badly distorted the magnified image even as they sharpened and brought into focus its detail.[7] In fact, the level of distortion was often so great as to preclude the compound microscope's usefulness over the single-lens instrument. As the microscopist C. R. Goring noted in 1824, by increasing the angle of aperture (or light incidence) on a compound microscope one could increase the detail visible on the specimen; however, as the angle of aperture increased, so did image distortion.[8] Malformation of the image thus was the price paid for detail and clarity.

The aberrant dual-lens instrument was brought into line with an improvement that effectively introduced yet another level of cultural mediation among the parts of the apparatus. Goring commissioned the production of a triple, apochromatic lens—a system designed to correct aberrations in the magnified and resolved image. The idea that a multiple lens system would function in a self-correcting manner was not new; what was new was his emphasis on the importance of light incidence in the definition of the image. By emphasizing the function of light in the formation of the image, Goring effectively suggested that light is not a natural presence in the image-making process but a physiological force that can distort the image and jam the apparatus. His contribution was to foreground the possibilities of strategically deploying light (by manipulating the lenses) to render the object studied.

The idea that lens and light both have agency and can be marshaled to render the object is crucial to the modern culture of microscopy. Long before techniques such as remote sensing or video surveillance were introduced in Western warfare and industry, compound microscopy effectively embodied the optical paradigms that would come to be associated with these late-twentieth-century techniques of discipline and domination. Like these later techniques, microscopy incorporated the individual observer in a decentralized and self-correcting virtual sensory apparatus—an apparatus capable of facilitating inspection of visually inaccessible territory with optical precision and detail. But as with these later techniques, a point of instability was always the lack of a reassuring view by eye of the territory charted. In the absence of a conventionally perceptible field, microscopists were burdened with the knowledge that what they saw through the viewfinder might still be a distortion—or, worse yet, an image artifact (a scratch in the surface of the lens or a stray fleck of dust).

In the absence of a conventional view, nineteenth-century microscope makers established optical standards to test the accuracy of their instruments. Interestingly, the standard against which they compared their views was not an object per se but a representation: a print rendered from the image viewed through the microscopic lens. In a reversal of the logic that would soon predominate in photography, an image became the standard or model for the human eye view. Goring, for example, adopted a group of natural objects (such as the wing of a moth), resolved them at different scales, and published enlarged photographic prints of these scales (figure 4.1).[9] Published in 1834, these images served as standards against which other microscopists could judge the accuracy of their own views of the same kind of moth. The idea was not that the microscopist could now be sure that his view of this kind of moth would be accurate, but rather that, if his instrument accurately registered this one class of object, it would accurately represent any object placed on its stage.

The introduction of the test object is significant because it suggests that from the early nineteenth century forward microscopists were more interested in verifying the accuracy of their instruments than in verifying the representational integrity of the microscopic scene they saw. It could be said that the primary focus of the scientific gaze in this context is the instrument itself and not the object viewed. Thus, long before Western artists and critical theorists engaged in reflexive interrogations of the technological apparatus, microscopists exhibited a modernist obsession with the means of production. But while it may be argued that this focus on the instrument was circumstantial (there being no available "promicroscopic" real), I would argue that this attention to the instrument is a symptomatic response to the unmanageability of the object.

Earlier I stated that the microscopic observer was subject to the corrective

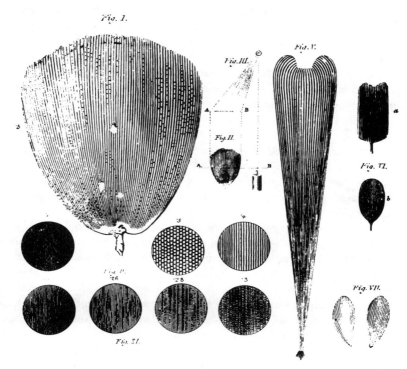

Figure 4.1. Goring's natural test objects. From Goring and Pritchard, *Micrographia*, plate II.

techniques of the instrument. I also noted that the object observed was managed and its image corrected. In Shaffer's analysis, discussed earlier, the object of the institutional gaze is celestial bodies, not human bodies. Shaffer, however, is rightfully concerned with the agency of workers subjected to managerial regulation of their acts of looking. Crary's focus is also the agency of human subjects and the regulation of their acts of looking. But by selecting physiological optics, Crary chose a reflexive field in which the object of the gaze is the observer's own body. This choice limits the analysis of power to the question of the subject of vision, the seeing subject. But the configuration of power is very different when the object of study is a human subject other than the observer, or when, as in microscopy, it is a body fragment or organic surrogate representing subjective human conditions such as health, sexuality, and even cultural identity. Recall that Watkins, in his microscopic experiments with the blood, argued that the physician can see pathology in the body prior to a person's subjective experience of symptoms. This claim is symptomatic of the real anxiety experienced by observers—the managerial subjects of the cultural institutions examined here—over the agency and au tonomy of their objects of study. In what follows, I attempt to uncover the agency of the object—its partial autonomy from the cultural institution that studies it; its subjectivity. The unseen "promicroscopic world" exists only in part as a phantasm of the Western viewing subject. It exists more significantly as a subjugated institutional history, a history of the agency of the object of the gaze, the subjective being represented in the bodily fragment posed on the microscopic stage.

The Unruly Objects of the Microscopic Gaze

What is most significantly subject to discipline within the cultural apparatus of microscopy is of course the object under surveillance—the specimen placed under the microscope, and the body from which it is derived or which it purports to represent. The development of microscopic test objects provides one example of the way in which the object studied (or the body it stands in for) is disciplined in microscopic culture. The regard of Goring's natural test objects provides a useful example of the way that the physical body, ostensibly microscopy's object of knowledge, is regarded with mistrust and even contempt. David Brewster, early photographer, author of publications on the stereoscope and natural magic, and inventor of the kaleidoscope, credited Goring's establishment of natural test objects (the moth wings) as the event that opened up the way for modern advances in microscopic lens systems.[10] However, as Turner points out, microscopists soon realized that physical variations within the same species made organic specimens unreliable test objects. The question was, which particular wing configuration was the true standard?[11] Noting that nature did not lend itself to the exactness of measurement demanded by science, the optician Friedrich Nobert proceeded to produce a mechanical norm against which to test the microscope's accuracy. Casting aside the organic test object, he used a machine called a circle engine to rule a set of imperceptibly fine lines on a glass specimen plate, mechanically ensuring that the distance between each line was exactly to his specifications. These carefully inscribed plates were then mounted on the microscope's stage, where the image was resolved and the distance between each groove carefully noted through the eyepiece. This measurement was then considered against Nobert's own figures to arrive at the exact degree of magnification. Nobert ruled plates with successively finer lines with the idea that numbers of lines resolved could be a gauge of instrument quality (figure 4.2).[12] These mechanical test objects were regarded as far more reliable than Goring's natural objects in the project of disciplining the instrument. Goring's microscopic moth images and Nobert's engraved micrometric standards verified the imaging instrument, and not the image or the eye of the observer. The status of the image of organic matter—what is

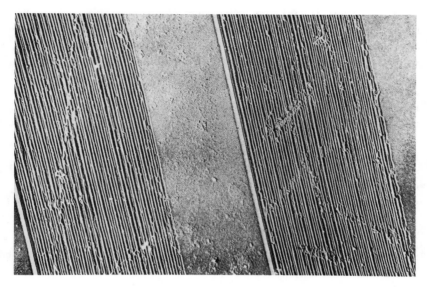

Figure 4.2. Nobert's mechanically ruled test plate. From G. L'E. Turner and S. Bradbury, "An Electron Microscopical Examination of Nobert's Finest Test-Plate of Twenty Bands," *Journal of the Royal Microscopic Society* 85 (1966): 441.

finally the microscopist's only area of contact with the actual entity under study—is finally judged on the basis of the status of the instrument. A mechanically produced object thus replaced the image of the living organism as the gauge of representational accuracy in microscopy.

Nobert's project expresses a more general mistrust of nature in microscopy. The "natural" eye, because it is subjective, cannot be depended upon to produce accurate representations. But, more importantly, the natural entity, because it is subjective and variable, is a deceptive representation even of its own properties. Mistrust of a dead moth's wings is an act of little apparent political consequence; however, it is important to recall that the moth wing is itself a placeholder for much more culturally loaded fragments of natural, organic matter. It stands in for drops of blood and sperm, bits of tissue, and the individual bodies and discrete pathologies and identities of which these fragments ostensibly are microcosms. The designation of organic test objects as unreliable visual sources is symptomatic of a broader mistrust of the natural body as an indicator even of its own conditions and states. Moreover, it is an unequivocal expression of technology's ascendancy as an uncontroverted agent in the production of the organic body. If bodily organs and viscera were exposed to examination in the eighteenth and early nineteenth centuries, they were quickly designated deceptive representatives of knowledge about the body. The machined test object was one response to this perceived deception. The machined object allowed the observer's focus to shift back to the instrument as the hoped-for site of trustworthy knowledge about the body. However, this movement did not entail a return to the camera-obscura mode of viewing, but signaled a new technological mode of visuality.

In the following section, I show how this principle functioned in the cinematic microscopic study of living systems. The films considered in the remainder of this chapter engage technologies and instruments of measurement that neither simply represent nor regulate nature, the organic body, and the subjects they so obliquely represent; they are privileged modes for generating new configurations of life and subjectivity that conform to the instrument. Forms of life that conform in advance to the conventions of microscopy are favored as test objects. And where living matter does not readily conform to these conventions, it is restructured to suit the means of study. The qualities of the cinematic microscopic, or the "cinemicroscopic," image are grafted back onto living matter, effectively manufacturing a new modernist conception of life.

The Cinemicroscopic Image: An Aesthetic of Flatness

Resolution standards such as the mechanically ruled plates made by Nobert were introduced essentially to measure distances across the image field. With a good microscope, one could easily compute the space between each ruled line on Nobert's test plate. But Nobert did not provide a means for measuring the depth of the grooves his machine carved. The microscopic view, like the photographic image, is essentially flat. However, unlike most photographs, the microscopic image does not represent potentially vast three-dimensional space on a flat field, but rather renders an already relatively shallow space. Despite this aesthetic of flatness, microscopic space in depth continually reasserted itself, returning to the image field only to be elided from the image. Even in contemporary microscopy, observers go to great lengths to manage depth, "cleaning up" and "correcting" unwanted levels of action in the microscopic frame.[13] My focus in this section, then, is the management of living matter—the scientific attempt to render the body and the perceived object in terms that conform to the instrument and its modes of representation.

In the nineteenth century, Marey strategically reduced the human body he studied to a series of lines and points, erasing those aspects of human physiology that interfered in the production of a graphic map of bodily movement. Like Marey, many later microscopists adapted their objects of study to the technique. For example, in a 1928 design for a cinemicroscopic apparatus for imaging the flow of blood in the capillaries in a living, intact body, two researchers at the hospital of the Rockefeller Institute for Medical Research in New York realized that their instrument would work only with relatively flat, translucent parts of the body. They chose to observe an extremely narrow area of tissue (the nail fold) in an already narrow appendage (the fingertip). Thus they effectively dispensed with the complexity of the corporeal body by selecting as its representative segment a structure that virtually exists in two dimensions. This penchant for flatness was symptomatic of a more pervasive cultural disavowal of the physical body as phantasm, as nightmarishly visceral and disorderly—a denial rationalized by a modernist demand for order, simplicity, particularity, and clarity. It might be said that microscopy was popularized in response to a general abhorrence and revulsion regarding the physical body in its complexity and depth—the very physical body that we see represented as a repulsive totality in the neurological films discussed in the previous chapter. By purging the familiar signifiers of corporeality from the body image, microscopy relieved itself of the need to address issues such as subjectivity, history, and identity so impossible to overlook in the type of image we saw in the neurological films. Moreover, by segmenting and slicing specimens taken from the actual body, microscopists incorporated outmoded techniques of corporal punishment into the scientific process, institutionalizing it in microcosm as a symbol of earlier modes of public discipline.

An aesthetic of abstraction that includes qualities such as flatness, segmentation, and planar division of space is not, of course, characteristic only of science. We see it in Western photography and painting during the first few decades of the twentieth century—in cubism, for example. The films considered in the following pages will be discussed as cubist texts. However, I will not be using the term "cubism" to refer only to an artistic movement embraced and forwarded by particular artists, nor will I suggest that personal influence or historical coincidence brought about a confluence of styles across art and science. Rather, I will argue that a "cubist" visual culture developed in part as a cultural response both to the epistemological instability of human observation and to the sight of the human body. The organic body and its anatomically explicit image, exposed in the previous century in all its visceral detail, is displaced by the notion of the body-in-process and its streamlined physiological time-image. I will attempt to show that the reverence for the flat and the abhorrence of dimensional form and the corporeal cannot be overlooked as operative forces in the formation of a pervasively cubist culture—a culture that reconfigures the bodily interior as an endlessly divisible series of flat surfaces and mobile networks.

The preference for test objects that conformed to the format of microscopy motivated researchers in their search for animal as well as human test objects. Frogs, for example, made ideal specimens, not only because they had relatively narrow appendages that fit relatively easily under the microscope, but because their translucent skin made their internal physiology readily visible under relatively low light levels. On the basis of this, the zoologist August Krogh used the frog as his test object for his important early cinematic studies of capillary action. Although Krogh specialized in zoology, he is well known for his contributions to human physiology. Like Marey and Muybridge, he applied his research to the study of respiration, exercise, and aviation physiology—areas with great applicability in industrial culture.[14] Krogh's early research focused on respiratory exchange through the lungs and skin. Though this work did not involve the use of images, it suggests a certain understanding of matter and form that helps to explain Krogh's later involvement in a "cubist" cinemicroscopy.

Krogh investigated with his laboratory partner (and wife) Marie Krogh whether oxygen was actively secreted from the lungs into the blood (the hypothesis of his mentor Christian Bohr) or whether it was transported by physical diffusion. The Kroghs found nothing to support the gas–secretion hypothesis, concluding that "the absorption of oxygen and the elimination of carbon dioxide in the lungs take place by diffusion and by diffusion alone. There is no trustworthy evidence of any regulation of this process on the part of the organism."[15] The diffusion hypothesis, then, indicates that the body does not fully regulate its own respiratory process but is subject to a chemical process that acts through it. This conceptual shift ascribes agency to what permeates the body (gases) rather than to the body's organs—a shift suggested in the terminological shift from "secretion," describing the action of the lungs upon gases, to "diffusion," describing the activity of gases spreading through the organism without the assistance of the lungs. The diffusion hypothesis suggests that the organs do not exist as fixed objects in "empty" space but are pervious entities. Organs such as the lungs are no longer understood to be organized according to distinctions of internal/external space or object/ground. They are no longer viewed as exercising control over the passage of matter through the body. Organs, including the skin, function less as boundaries than as permeable, overlapping screens of planar space.

The diffusion experiment was conducted in 1909, a year after the first painterly "experiments" of Georges Braque identified retrospectively with the origins of cubism. The spatial conventions developed in Braque's early cubist paintings have much in common with the Kroghs' diffusion hypothesis. Most significant is Braque's interest in analyzing "negative" space—the area between objects in a still life, for example. "What most attracted me," Braque later explained, "and what was the governing principle of cubism, was the materialization of this new space I sensed."[16] It can be said that the Kroghs also sensed the materialization of a new space when they recognized the agency of gas as it moved between organs, the "objects" of their "still life," as it were. Just as Braque viewed space as having materiality and hence pictorial agency, so the Kroghs saw gas as having a previously unrecognized agency in the mechanics of life. In Krogh's work, this recognition of agency in a force moving within the body is a source of anxiety, generating a desire to intervene and regulate.

August Krogh himself made a connection between the materiality of bodily gases and the substantiality of pictorial space when in 1920 he produced *Blood Circulation in the Frog*,[17] a microscopic film study of capillary circulation. The film shows a cross-sectional view of blood flow in the capillaries. If the diffusion hypothesis stressed the agency and relative autonomy of the movement of an entity through the "negative" space of the body, this film is evidence of a certain anxiety about the freedom of that flow. Shots depicting "normal" capillary flow in the frog's bladder (figure 4.3) are followed by sequences showing the flow's change in response to chemical and mechanical stimuli. Krogh charges the frog's body with an electrical current, prods it with needles, and injects it with chemicals, carefully noting in intertitles the variation in the rate of flow introduced by each intervention. The film concludes with Krogh physically blocking the blood flow. The moving image of the corpuscles slowing to a halt is an image that calibrates death, allowing the viewer to chart with precision the time and rate of the process of dying.

Krogh's film study is at once clinically distant and deadly horrific. He employs traditional codes of scientific omniscience, distancing his viewers from the living object, its mutilation and potential pain, and the presence of his own hand in the process. The body (that of the frog, that of the researcher) is elided from the image; we are presented with an abstract clinical view of corpuscles in close-up. The film is finally nothing more than tedious to all but the professional observer invested in its data and findings. Yet in this coolly indifferent presentational style is depicted a narrative of cruelty made all the more stunning by its apparent dullness: Krogh electrifies, prods, poisons, and finally kills his object.

Although the object in question is a frog, and Krogh's treatment of it routine in scientific research, it is important to recall that the laboratory animal is a surrogate for the human body—a convenient site for the performance of acts that would be deemed sadistic and transgressive if performed on the human body. This laboratory visual culture is, after all, a culture of human corporeal supervision and discipline, even in cases where the human body is not directly studied. For certainly disciplining of the subject need not entail physical contact with the body, but is more often effected through intermediate sites. The animal body is a symbolic site where human corporeal regulation is carried out.

The obliteration of bodily presence and the signifiers of pain from the image field is not unique to microscopy. Foucault writes that at the beginning of the nineteenth century, "the great spectacle of physical punishment disappeared; the tortured body was avoided; the theatrical representation of pain was excluded from punishment."[18] Here, in 1920, we see a peculiar

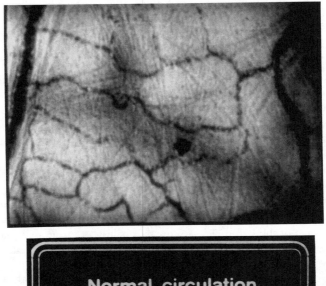

Figure 4.3. Frames from Krogh's *Blood Circulation in the Frog* (1920).

mutation of the repressed spectacle of public torture. The institutional punishment of the body through the ritual infliction of pain is displaced from the public theater of the streets to the private stage of the laboratory microscope. In the laboratory setting, acts of punishment are legitimated (they are in the service of knowledge about human life and health) and neutralized (they are rendered a routine part of laboratory culture). In the laboratory, ritual practice is "cleaned up" and designated as technique; subjective factors like the hand of the researcher or the experience of the test object are omitted from the representation. The infliction of pain is incorporated into institutional practice as a privatized ritual knowledge, its effects elided from the broader social scene.

Although the image of the shocked, prodded, and poisoned frog is rendered an artifact of mundane laboratory routine, the object—the frog's circulation—nonetheless emerges as an unstable element in this clean system. In the published analysis of the experiment, we find all manner of techniques used to manage the flow of blood. Krogh and his coauthor Rehberg present frame enlargements, scales of magnification, and textual analysis of both. Not only do they compare successive shots and frames of blood flow under the same magnification; they measure and account for variations in its rate of speed due to differences in magnification.[19] Indeed, even camera speed is accounted for in the attempt to calibrate the subjective conditions of both instrument and flow.[20] Yet the movement of blood resisted containment in at least one respect: it refused to move only in the lateral dimension, flowing instead into the depth of the image, in three-dimensional space. This posed serious problems for Krogh since, like Nobert's test plates, his instrument did not account for movement in any direction other than laterally. How he managed the factor of movement in depth provides some insight into his regard for the physicality of the complete, dimensional body.

As has been noted, Krogh had already chosen a relatively flat, translucent organism, the frog. His next step was to isolate an even flatter part of the body: he drew the frog's tongue out of its mouth and pinned it down flat across the microscope stage. But although he had secured a flat entity in an already flat body, he was still confounded by depth of field in the image itself:

> At low magnification the depth of focus is a disturbing factor and in the picture, which shows the pulsation of the main artery of the tongue, the bands of striped muscle running across the vessels have a somewhat disturbing effect. On the whole experience points to the conclusion that in microkinematography the best results are obtained at high magnifications.[21]

In Krogh's view, high magnifications give the best results not because they provide greater information about the specimen but because they eliminate depth of field. The "disturbing effect" Krogh refers to is the occurrence of action in depth throughout the specimen's body—for example, bands of muscle overlapping the main artery and thereby hiding it. By increasing magnification in the microscope lens (the camera lens being removed), Krogh limited depth in the focal field, in effect eliminating from view the bands of muscle that blocked his view of the blood. It is as if the body is deceptive, even transgressive, simply because it has depth and complexity. Bodily depth causes "disturbances" in the image field; thus the body must be corrected (rendered flat) by the microscope. Cubism, in this context, becomes a technique for disciplining the unruly dimensional body.

Pictorial photography and cinematography both situate objects in three-dimensional space by using reflected light, relying on lenticular perspective and cues such as overlap and internal modulation of objects, relative size of known objects, and the like to constitute a continuous space. But cinemicrography, as we have seen, sought to eliminate these spatial cues (by eliminating the camera lens, for example). As the introduction of panchromatic film required less intense (incandescent) lighting in the film industry, similarly the relatively lower light levels on the microscopic stage made it necessary to open up the camera diaphragm, reducing the potential depth of field to a minimum.[22] Indeed, by removing the camera lens altogether, both perspectival space and a centralized viewpoint could be eliminated from the process.

If not according to conventions such as perspective, object/space oppositions, and overlap, how was this flat optical field organized? What was its historical context? Flatness in microscopy closely matches the condition of flatness in late cubist paintings described by the art critic Clement Greenberg. According to Greenberg, flatness is a "disembodied attribute and expropriated property detached from everything not itself."[23] In other words, depth and object/ground relations in cubist space finally refer to spatial conventions themselves, rather than to the objects they ostensibly represent.[24] In the following passage Greenberg offers a take on cubism's relationship to its object. Interestingly, the metaphor he uses is a familiar object of cinemicroscopic analysis:

> Cubism undertook a completely two-dimensional transcription of three-dimensional phenomena. . . . The world was stripped of its surface, of its skin, and the skin was spread flat on the flatness of the picture plane.[25]

This unpeeling of the voluminous folds of physical surfaces is most evident in the flatness of synthetic cubist painting, where the modulated surface that renders volume is peeled and flattened in a spatially aberrant image, bearing the distortion so familiar in contour maps of the world. Interestingly, Krogh also had a technique for making spherical specimens into surfaces. Taking dimensional objects like a frog's distended bladder, he would affix a cover sheet to the body, flattening the protrusion to create a surface parallel to the focal plane of the lens. Represented as a succession of flat surfaces, the microscopic body was transformed into a series of light-penetrable sheets even before it was placed on the microscopic stage.

A modality that takes this paradigm to its limits is described by the historian of science Antony Michaelis. This is the serial section film, in which physical matter (a tumor, a piece of tissue) is sliced with a microtome, an instrument used for cutting microscopically thin specimens. The cross-sectional segments are affixed in succession onto the frames of a strip of film. This strip is then rephotographed and projected. Michaelis describes a project of 1907 in which a researcher composed a film from two thousand successive cross-sections of a brain specimen which, when projected, provided a virtual tour that passed its viewers through a previously impenetrable mass. In the same year, another researcher published a description of a similar project in which he did not photograph the serial slices, but simply projected the original film onto which the sections were affixed, much as Braque pasted actual pieces of wood-grain wallpaper to the surface of his canvas instead of simulating wood with paint. Projected, this film simulated movement perpendicularly through the dense structure of the object with much the same effect as a camera moving through a foggy indeterminate space in which atmospheric particles scatter light diffusely across the field.[26]

Whereas in Krogh's film deep space is carefully elided, serial section films use the same principle of planar abstraction to render the body a deep space that viewers may tour. But here space functions as an abstract representation of matter. If Krogh and Braque dissolved the object/ground dichotomy by affirming that gas and atmosphere have materiality, these films ensured that objects would be regarded as themselves composed of permeable matter. In the serial section film, movement also plays a purely representational role. Filmic "movement" through the sectioned object does not represent actual movement through a space; rather, it represents static volume. Whereas in cubist paintings planar surfaces replace more conventional techniques for rendering depth, such as overlap, perspectival composition, and foreshortening, here movement represents depth. Each successive frame presents a part of the object in the immediate foreground of the image field. Like Krogh's physical and optical isolation of individual planes, cross-sectioning renders the specimen pervious to light, giving each frame the characteristics of a dense, "foggy" field rather than that of a "negative" space containing solid objects. The viewer visually seeps into the object, not so much penetrating as visually infusing it (recall Krogh's diffusion hypothesis). Distinctions of interior/exterior space, object/ground, and viewing space / screen space are dissolved in this viewing experience. Like the textural surfaces of late cubist paintings, serial section space is constituted nonpictorially as a dense surface or screen. No compositional cues direct the eye to any unitary object or point.

In an account that is useful if only for its reductive characterization, John Golding summarizes cubism as an art movement that

> had evolved a completely original, antinaturalistic kind of figuration, which had at the same time stripped bare the mechanics of pictorial creation, and had in the process gone a long way toward destroying artificial barriers between abstraction and representation.[27]

In the set of films to which I will now turn, we see exactly this kind of "antinaturalistic" figuration of the organic and this destruction of the division between abstraction and representation. During the 1930s, U.S. anatomists Elliot Round Clark and Eleanor Linton (or, as *Men of Science* would have it,

"Mrs. E. R.") Clark developed a cubist apparatus that dissolved distinctions not only between object and field and between abstraction and representation, but between life and instrument. Implanting in their test animals (rabbits) what they called a "virtual test-tube in vivo," they filmed what they understood to be a natural process in the living body. But here nature is made over to resemble nothing more closely than a two-dimensional film fully incorporated within the body.

Donna Haraway, in her well-known cyborg manifesto, notes that contemporary science fiction and modern medicine are both full of cyborgs, "creatures simultaneously animal and machine, who populate worlds ambiguously natural and crafted."[28] In the project I am about to describe, the Clarks seem to regard their technologically altered rabbits' ears as cyborg sites—as, to borrow Haraway's words, "couplings between organism and machine, each conceived as coded devices, in an intimacy and with a power that was not generated in the history of sexuality."[29] The Clarks created a living system for reproduction out of a joining of the organic and the technological. In doing so, they also contributed to the creation of new technological mythologies about reproduction in a postgender world—a myth for scientists in the first half of the century that fueled the pervasive mythology of the late-twentieth-century scientist as technician of the postsexual laboratory reproduction of human life.

Implanting the Cinema in Nature

The Clarks began research in embryology as students of the American anatomist Franklin P. Mall at Johns Hopkins. Early in his career, Mall had trained with the noted German experimental physiologist Carl Ludwig.[30] Although the Clarks, like Mall, held positions in the field of anatomy, their methodology was grounded in experimental physiology and instrumentation. From its earliest stages, their work was concerned with human physiology—the living systems found in organic matter that can be studied to learn about human life.

Like the Kroghs, the Clarks initially selected the tadpole, an animal with a conveniently transparent tail, as their model for studies in physiology. It was their mission to widen their scope to "higher animals" in the hope of applying their findings more directly to human anatomy and physiology. However, no natural transparent region that suited their means of study was available in the body of the live mammal and, like Krogh and others, they were not inclined to change their means of study. Instead, they surgically produced the condition of transparency in the living body of the mammal of their choice, the rabbit. Not only did they breed a colony of rabbits suitable in size and disposition to their purposes; they surgically altered the animals so that their bodies would exactly suit their techniques of observation.

One need only recall Nobert's objections to the use of natural test objects to understand the Clarks' perceived need for an isolated, uniform, and easily reproducible research colony. Rabbits were appealing to scientists because they bred prolifically and were regarded as having a natural inclination to docility. If the object of science can be said to be the regulation of human bodies, the tractable body of the rabbit might be regarded as an ideal model for human experimentation. By breeding animals in colonies, researchers gained a high level of control over the kinds of characteristics that predominated in a given community. Using the techniques of animal husbandry, scientists encouraged the reproduction of characteristics and qualities suited to particular experiments. Certain characteristics regarded as generally favorable (such as docility or thin coats) could thus be bred to become a norm within a particular colony. As with microscopic test objects, test animals were designed to provide an infrastructural norm. The idea of a general state of the species in nature introduced a disturbing degree of subjective variation (as we saw with the use of the moth wing as a test object); but this idea of a general norm in the colony proved to be less easily obtainable than, for example, mechanically produced test objects.

In her study of the production of animals as research materials, historian Adele E. Clarke relates the words of the head of a major zoology laboratory seeking funds for a vivarium, a facility for housing live test animals: "The study of living animals has replaced to a considerable extent the study of their dead bodies, and a vivarium is as much a need of the modern zoological laboratory as a museum."[31] This pronouncement of 1914 echoes Charcot's heralding of the Salpêtrière in 1862 as a museum of living pathology. The vivarium is just such a living museum; however, in the vivarium typologies are not just observed; they are, quite literally, bred. Whereas Charcot and his colleagues believed themselves to be observing pathological processes as they occurred spontaneously in the bodies of their charges, the Clarks deliberately generated pathological and other kinds of processes in the bodies of the colonies they produced. In the following passage, they describe at length their attempts to generate a particular kind of body, while insisting that the body they produced is above all a normal state of the species. Their account is striking in its identification of the conventions of human domestic culture, and especially maternal caregiving, as key elements in the production of a docile rabbit "family" able to accept subjection to laboratory testing as a routine part of its daily life:

> We have found it decidedly worth while to raise our own rabbits, in order to secure the healthiest large-eared stock, and to gentle them and accustom them to being handled, since such animals remain quiet and normal throughout observa-

tion. In this connection we cannot refrain from commending the extremely faithful work of Mrs. Larry Bentz, whose devoted service in the care and raising of the animals has played no small part in the success of our studies. Rabbits which are healthy and free from external parasites soon grow quite accustomed to the animal board; they lie for hours without struggling, and give every appearance of being comfortable and at ease, i.e., they lie quite still, with relaxed muscles, quiet moderate breathing, and normal circulation. . . . They remain in perfect health, are plump and active, and have smooth, glossy fur after being kept on the board for five to eight hours a day for four months or more. In fact, there are now several rabbits with chambers which have been in place more than twelve months, which have been placed on the board for observation perhaps 200 times, and which are in perfect health. Apparently, they learn to accept the procedure as a normal part of their existence.[32]

Interestingly, the authors understand a "normal" condition to be any condition to which the animal may be enculturated, and not the animal's condition "in nature." Physiological mechanisms of adaptation and their effects on the overall life of the animal are elided from the picture. The Clarks do not mention the possibility of more subtle signs of trauma or fear (for example, a potential analgesic response to pain). Furthermore, the generation of an ideal test colony did not stop with the enculturation of a community that experienced such things as surgical intervention and extensive surveillance as part of routine daily life. The Clarks literally retooled their animals' bodies and habits to make them conform to experimental procedures. For example, in an attempt to render a part of the rabbit body more easily observable under the microscope, they physically implanted an instrument for observing growth within the living ear. This device, which they called a window, was surgically implanted in a hole cut through one ear.[33] This window on physiology comprised two layers of celluloid separated by a microscopically thin space. Metal fittings bound the plastic panels at the edges of the surgical wound, blocking tissue growth over the outer surfaces of the celluloid. Blood vessels and cells actively grew within the celluloid walls of the window, extending out from the margins of the circular wound. The viewer-friendly ear chamber was conveniently small, fitting neatly under the microscope to afford the Clarks and their research associates a custom-made window on living physiology (figures 4.4 and 4.5).[34]

The ear chambers in no way functioned for the Clarks as reproductions or simulations of living processes; rather, they were regarded as areas of actual, "normal" physiological growth. But the fact that this "normal" growth bore little similarity to other aspects of the rabbit's biological body is clear in the case of the Clarks' regard of the property of permeability in the celluloid window. The celluloid sheets used to seal the chamber were, like the skin itself, permeable. Permeability is a vital property in capillary exchange. This fact would suggest that celluloid shared a property of tissue, and therefore

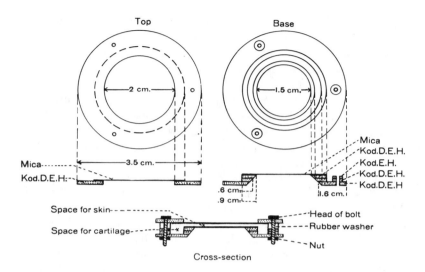

Figure 4.4. Diagram of Clark rabbit-ear chamber.

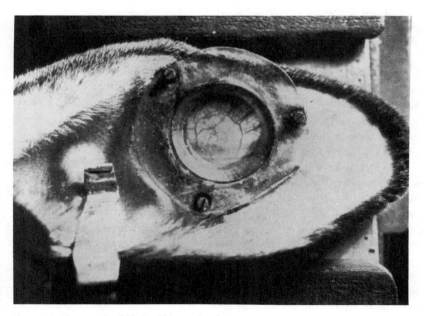

Figure 4.5. Photograph of Clark rabbit-ear chamber.

would be suitable to the project. However, because the celluloid sheet was permeable, growth took place not only in the chamber, but on the outer surface of the "window." In other words, the bodily depth repressed in the experimental apparatus resurfaced as a "problem" in technique. Rather than seeing this tendency of growth to take place on more than one plane as an indication of the routine nature of the process, the Clarks saw it as an annoyance precisely because it prohibited their observation of a single, reduced layer of growth laterally. Like Krogh, they wanted a single plane in the image field. They replaced the tissuelike celluloid with glass and mica sheets, impermeable substances that sealed off the inner environment of the chamber from the passage of everything except light.[35]

The Clarks described the transparent chamber as "a virtual test-tube in vivo";[36] they referred to the growth of tissue within the thin space between the two celluloid sheets as a "growth in two dimensions."[37] Not only was the visual instrument fused directly into the live subject; the subject was mechanically adapted to generate its own two-dimensional surface. The physiological process was a result of both the tissue growth in the animal and the determination of that growth by the visual apparatus fused with the body. This is not to say that the rabbit was mechanized, or that life was imputed to the visual apparatus, but that this technique established a critical continuity between human physiology and its technological prostheses. The technologies implanted in the animal to better observe it were now considered integral parts of the "normal" body and "normal" physiological processes under study.[38]

Within a few years of the development of these test tubes in vivo, the Clarks began to make microscopic motion picture films shot through these rabbit-ear windows.[39] Like Krogh's project, these films were used to measure blood circulation under different conditions. In the 1933 reel *Effects of Heat and Cold on Blood Circulation*, the scale introduced in the frame is not a scale of magnification (as in Krogh's films) but of temperature. First is shown "normal circulation" at 78 degrees Fahrenheit. This, intertitles explain, is followed by "local application of snow" (note the choice of naturalist terminology to describe what is in fact an ice pack). The process is reversed as the room is heated to above 100 degrees. A final title reads, "Observation showed increased circulation following the application of heat, with evidence of increased diffusion through the vessel wall," concluding with the assurance that the rabbits have experienced "no harmful effects whatsoever" (figure 4.6).

Like Krogh, the Clarks were concerned with measurements of speed laterally across the two-dimensional field only; however, because they had profilmically eliminated depth in the body itself, they did not have to contend as much with limiting depth in the image. In effect, the windows were a virtual film in themselves, insofar as they made visible the movement of tissue growth in a framed two-dimensional field. The Clarks nonetheless introduced all manner of measurement techniques to manage their object. In

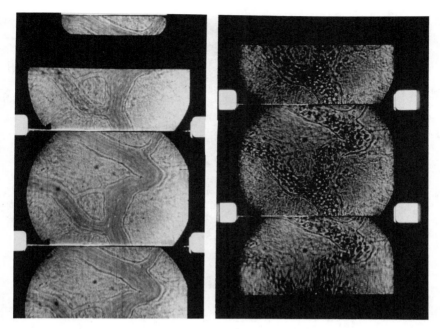

Figure 4.6. Frames from a Clark film demonstrating effects of heat (left) and cold (right) on blood circulation (1933).

their essays about the film studies, they used microscopic camera lucida drawings made from a few hours to a few months apart: these are presented, like frame enlargements, in series to depict growth over time. Frame enlargements and still photomicrographs are also included in the essays. Numerical data derived through a micrometer eyepiece are represented by charts. Thus, a single process is rendered in the form of tables, line graphs, serial drawings, and film frames (figures 4.7 and 4.8).[40] Clearly, if the microscope is an instrument for correcting and calibrating the perception of the object, it is only a part of an even more heterogeneous technology, one that incorporates a wide range of regimes of vision and techniques of analysis. The implications of this scene for the observer are by now clear; but what of the object? More specifically, what was the object of the Clarks' study of the surgically manufactured windows on physiology?

Wound as Womb

The Clarks make an interesting observation about their own technique. They explain that although the surgeon would refer to the sealed hole in the ear as a wound, the pathologist would regard it as a process of repair:

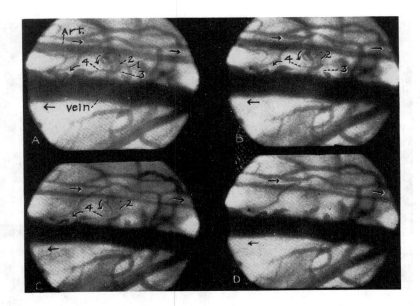

Figure 4.7. Film frames as they appear in a published analysis of growth taking place in the Clark rabbit-ear chamber.

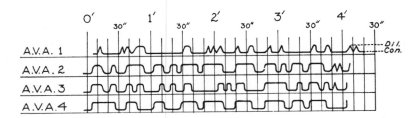

Figure 4.8. Graph of growth taking place in the four frames of the Clark rabbit-ear chamber.

> Doubtless the pathologist would prefer such terms as "repair" and "late stages of aseptic inflammation" to describe the phenomena observed, while the surgeon would use the term "wound healing." Such differences in nomenclature for the same processes only serve to emphasize the importance of the method for investigations of problems in many different fields of biology and medicine.[41]

Although they do not deny the value of their method to medicine and surgery, the Clarks maintain that its use in a variety of fields is highly subjective. Furthermore, they argue that their implanted windows are instances of pathology only in a few cases—instances where infection sets in, or where the chamber is rejected by the ear. Clearly, they lack interest in the regard of their project in pathology and medicine; however, their approach precludes recognition of a pathological condition as such where most other fields could not fail to acknowledge its presence.[42] Theirs is a remarkable transposition of notions of pathology and life. They regard the window-wound they engineer as a normal site of life in the broadest and most paradigmatic of senses:

> It is chiefly because of the exact resemblance of the process of vascular invasion and subsequent differentiation under the conditions present in these windows in the rabbit's ear to the early process of vessel growth as it takes place in the embryo that we have used such anatomical and cytological designations as "new growth of blood vessels" for the processes described.[43]

The ear wound/window is presented as a paradigm for embryological growth; for the Clarks, it represents the evolution of life itself. Indeed, the ear of the rabbit is conceived as an adequate model for the female body in general, the site of embryonic growth in the mammal: "The process corresponds in all essentials to the process of early growth of blood vessels in the embryo," they assert.[44] The wound is transformed into a womb, situated within the ear of the rabbit. Research on the development of the embryo is thus displaced onto a scientifically engineered wound, a region conveniently reconfigured to facilitate viewing and to stand in for the female reproductive organs. The motion picture film becomes one in a series of screen images among the many "films" (of tissue, of capillary walls) that make up this new narrative of biological reproduction.

Conclusion

If subjugated knowledges are the "historical contents that have been buried and disguised in a functionalist coherence of formal systematization,"[45] cinemicroscopy, analyzed here in a few particular instances, performs in a quite literal way this kind of disguising and systematizing of bodies—and of the lives and subjectivities encoded in them. Like the cause of epilepsy, history and knowledge of the object of the scientific gaze is thought to lie "far below par," disguised by the conceptual schema that abstracts the corporeal body into a formal system, a planar cubist text. As we see in the Clark films, what is concealed in the flat microscopic text is the status of the microscopic image as a microcosm of cultural norms about the body and subjectivity, a system in which a pathological condition (a wound) may represent anything from normal health to normal "living, growing" bodies. The history of the subject that is truly rendered invisible in this microscopic world is finally not a history of the seeing subject, but a history of the social subject whose body is diced, sliced, replaced by user-friendly animal and machine surrogates, or interspersed with technological mechanisms, only to be magnified and resolved beyond any hope of recognition or restitution. But should we lament the loss of this organic body? Is there a more useful reading of the dynamics within the capillary techniques of power? To speak to these questions, I return for a moment to Haraway's concept of the cyborg.

The organic body—the one decomposed, splayed, and reconfigured by the techniques I describe in this book—is the mythical Western humanist body, the full, contained body of the unitary subject. Haraway's cyborg myth is contradictory and perverse because it encompasses both this body in its most exaggerated form and a transcendence of this body. The cyborg is both "the awful apocalyptic telos of the 'West's' escalating dominations of abstract individuation, an ultimate self"[46] and the regeneration of this monster as something other than our enemy, as perhaps our potentiality, in a postgender, postorganic, posttechnophobic world.[47] The embryonic life the Clarks generate in the rabbit may be a minor prehistoric tale in the narrative of reproductive engineering. But might it not also be read as a prescient gesture toward postsexual modes of reproduction, and toward a body that goes beyond the dictates of ideologies of the natural and the organic?

CHAPTER 5

Decomposing the Body:
X Rays and the Cinema

To MANY FILM HISTORIANS, 1895 is the year of the "birth" of the cinema; for historians of technology and medicine, however, 1895 is the year of the discovery of the X ray. This chapter takes up the historical convergence of the cinema and radiography. In previous chapters, my focus has been intrainstitutional production and uses of films in medical science. My intention was to provide an analysis of laboratory discourse and culture. With this chapter, I begin to give closer attention to the reception of the moving X ray in the broader culture. As an imaging technique, the X-ray image lent itself to all manner of public interpretations, meanings, and fantasies, generating a vociferous public response that earned the designation "X-ray mania." X-ray images functioned, and continue to function, as icons, fetishes, and artifacts of health, life, sexuality, and, most significantly, death. In the following pages, I consider X-ray technology as a pervasive and perverse cultural apparatus—one that confounds the distinctions between the public and the private; specialized knowledge and popular fantasy; and scientific discourse, high art, and popular culture. As an aesthetic and a set of conventions, the X-ray is both gothic and modernist; as a medical tool, it has been regarded as a technique for both destroying and saving lives; and as a mode of scientific knowledge, it has revealed more about the modern body than any other imaging modality, drawing on both centuries-old iconography and modern visual paradigms to generate new configurations of the body.

Finally, the X ray is a major technique of twentieth-century medical knowledge and power. It has been a war machine, used in national battles against disease and in battles for global prominence in science; and it also has been a metaphorical site of major importance. The X-rayed body, stripped of its overinscribed gender- and race-encoded epidermis and organs, is an apt figure both for the nightmare of eugenics, with its agenda of eradicating some body types, and for utopian fantasies of a social order no longer predicated on typologies on the organic body. As precursor and prototype of the new contemporary imaging modalities that have flooded the medical scene since midcentury, and as the most institutionally pervasive and heavily subsidized diagnostic imaging technique of the twentieth century, the X ray is the pivotal site of investigation for this book's exploration of medicine's technological/visual knowledge, desire, and power. It is also the most conflicted site, embodying multiple paradigms of visuality and multiple political agendas.

In the sections that follow, I begin by reconsidering some of the origin myths of the X ray. I reread radiography's prehistory in order to reinscribe there the bodies of researcher and test subject, and in order to reconfigure a history that has been dominated by technological determinism. I first consider the perverse spectatorial pleasure of X-ray researchers and the public confronted with the static X-ray photograph. Here we find an extreme example of a technique that renders its viewing subject an object of a pervasive disciplinary gaze—a truly radiant gaze—that threatens to perform a quite literal disintegration of the body. I then turn to the X-ray motion picture, considering its place among the cultures of U.S. literary and art-world modernism, and its status as a popular image and technique of medical authority over life, sexuality, and death. The analysis of X-ray research films that concludes this chapter raises questions about the interdependency of art and science in the construction of a modernist culture; more importantly, though, it makes clear the centrality of popular memory and visual spectacle in the disciplinary techniques of scientific modernism. The X-ray motion picture ultimately reconstructs the surfaces, flesh and blood, and depth of the humanist body that are so dramatically stripped away in, for example, the microscopic image or the static X-ray photograph. In doing so, the X-ray film breathes life into a system of visual knowledge that has made good, more than any other technique, the threat of corporeal annihilation metaphorically posed by medical imaging in other contexts. If the modernist techniques described in the previous chapter introduce a new model of organic-technological life, the X-ray motion picture responds to that futuristic promise by reinvesting the abstract body image with all of the pictorial conventions of the full, natural body. The X-ray body is rendered with organ-surfaces and blood; it is invested with a synchronized voice; and finally, it is treated with the popular 1950s technique of 3-D associated with science fiction film (and its image of outer space), rendering the body's inner space a place of futuristic fantasies.

This chapter focuses primarily on the subjectivity of the radiologist, and the place of the X ray in research practices. But, as this chapter begins to suggest, the X-ray image has been crucial in the shaping of public perceptions of life, health, and the body. In my concluding chapter, I consider the representation and agency of women in the public health campaign to eradicate tuberculosis, a campaign that used both X rays and the motion picture in interrelated ways. Although women's bodies are constructed as aberrant sites, sites that harbor disease and resist diagnostic methods, women also are granted a privileged status as agents in the work of community disease surveillance and treatment. In this final chapter I foreground most fully the crucial issue of agency on the part of those living "objects" of the disciplinary gaze.

Taming the Pathological Ray (Decomposing Origin Tales)

The histories of the X ray and the cinema coincide in concrete and matter-of-fact ways. The Lumières and Thomas Edison, designated "fathers" of the cinema, experimented with X-ray-sensitive emulsions within months of the publication of physicist Wilhelm Conrad Roentgen's discovery that X rays could produce images of the skeletal system. Edison promoted the X-ray in popular demonstrations much as he promoted the cinema, publicly announcing in 1896 that he would soon be able to image the brain through the human skull. Though his attempts were never successful (it will shortly become clear why), they were nonetheless surrounded by a media blitz that placed Edison at center stage in the popular frenzy over the "new rays" and their deathly skeletal images.

The focus of these cinema industrialists and inventors on the X ray indicates that there were high hopes for the technique's marketability, and especially for its viability as a popular media form. Yet, despite the mania over the rays that swept the West at the turn of the century, X-ray imaging never emerged as a medium of popular culture like the cinema. Rather, it remained a specialized scientific-medical process, though a highly lucrative one. The following passage, taken from a *Journal of the American Medical Association* article of 1903, provides some clues as to why the X-ray image never gained the status of entertainment media:

> At this somewhat late day, Mr. Edison, and through him, the newspapers have all of a sudden discovered that x-rays can cause injuries, and, like many other belated discoveries, the topic is now one of lively interest in the daily press. According to the various newspaper reports, Mr. Edison's injuries are interesting. His left eye is out of focus, his digestion is upset, and lumps have formed all through the region of his stomach. He knows it is the result of the x-rays because he held the tube close to his stomach when he was working with the x-rays five or six years ago. The disease from which he is suffering is of a most interesting character, and no doctor is able to tell him anything about it; he ought to have been able to find out, for among the many specialists he has consulted there is one man who has dissected more than four thousand bodies, and if a man who has made four thousand dissections can not tell you what is the cause of lumps in your body, who can?[2]

The *Journal of the American Medical Association* entry remarks that Edison's findings regarding his strange afflictions are rather late in coming. It does not mention that the findings have come too late to save Clarence Dally, Edison's assistant in his earliest X-ray investigations, who, by 1903, had already been afflicted with an X-ray-caused cancer so invasive that his limbs had to be amputated, joint by joint, in an attempt to check its spread. The link between X rays and cancer was unmistakable. Dally's cancer originated in the hand that he repeatedly passed under the Edison fluoroscope to test its function. Dally and his boss were in fact keenly aware long before 1903 that a correlation existed between the rays and bodily damage. Dally found lesions and sores on the exposed hand soon after his earliest experiments with the fluoroscope. Yet he persisted in his experiments even after he became aware that the inflammations were cancerous. When one hand became ulcerated and unusable, he subjected his other hand to the same repeated tests, only to repeat the same gruesome experience. Dally died of X-ray-induced carcinoma in 1904 after undergoing multiple amputations.[3]

 I relate this tale to emphasize that the X ray was not simply an imaging technique. It was also a force that caused real physiological effects in the body. This fact was not lost on early researchers, who tried to develop the X-ray apparatus as a therapeutic device. What drove Edison, Dally and other scientists to pursue a technology that demonstrated so clearly its potential for bodily destruction and death was not only the thrill of seeing the deathly spectacle of the skeletal system but also the potential to harness the physiological force of the ray as a medical treatment—that is, as radiation therapy. The masochism of Dally and many others was rationalized in part by their insistence that the rays that caused burns and cancers in their bodies could both identify (through images) and heal pathologies in the body.[4]

Some early researchers anthropomorphized the X ray, investing it with a moral imperative to wipe out disease. For example, an account discussing the X ray's therapeutic use, written in the same year as the report on Edison's strange symptoms, claims that X rays exhibit a selective "predilection" for "cells out of place," targeting and dissolving aberrant growths on the skin's surface.[5] However, the X ray was more often represented during these years as a wild, unknown natural force that had to be harnessed and managed in order to be put to good use. Thus the early history of X-ray imaging is not only about the management and control of bodies through imaging; it is also about the management and domestication of a potentially dangerous force of nature in medical culture. Hence I begin my analysis of origin myths with an account of the taming of the ray.

In chapter 2, I briefly considered the astronomer François Arago's regard of the photograph as a measure of light intensity. For Arago, the daguerreotype was in part a reflexive index of light intensity. However, scientists had other techniques to measure and quantify light intensity. This was not the case with the X ray. The photographic image functioned as the primary indicator of the X ray's very existence. Much as the microscopic view functioned as proof of the existence of entities that could not be perceived by the eye, the X-ray image was the first indication of the existence of a natural force whose source was unknown (hence the designation "X"). As the following account makes clear, Roentgen's most significant "discovery" was a technique for producing images, and not a "natural" force. I quote at length from this memorial speech delivered at the British Roentgen Society two years after Roentgen's discovery because it is a good example of the construction of science's history as a series of moments of blinding truth, brilliant male visions, and revelations of nature:

> November the eighth, 1895, will ever be memorable in the history of Science. On that day a light which, so far as human observation goes, never was on land or sea, was first observed. The observer, Prof. Wilhelm Conrad Röntgen. The place, the Institute of Physics at the University of Würzburg in Bavaria. What he saw with his own eyes, a faint flickering greenish illumination upon a bit of cardboard, painted over with a fluorescent chemical preparation. Upon the faintly luminous surface a dark line of shadow. All this in a carefully darkened room, from which every known kind of ray had been scrupulously excluded. In that room a Crookes tube, stimulated internally by sparks from an induction coil, but carefully covered by a shield of black cardboard, impervious to every known kind of light, even the most intense. Yet in the darkness, expressly arranged so as to allow the eye to watch for luminous phenomena, nothing visible until the hitherto unrecognized rays, emanating from the Crookes tube and penetrating the cardboard shield, fell upon the luminescent screen, thus revealing their existence and making darkness visible. From seeing the illumination by the invisible rays of a fluorescent screen, and the line of shadow across it, the work of tracing back that shadow to the object which caused it, and of verifying the source of the rays to be the Crookes tube, was to the practiced investigator but the work of a few minutes. The invisible rays—for they were invisible save when they fell on the painted screen—were found to have a penetrative power hitherto unimagined. They penetrated cardboard, wood and cloth with ease. They would even go through a thick plank, or a book of 2000 pages, lighting up the screen placed on the other side. But metals such as copper, iron, lead, silver and gold were less penetrable, the densest of them being practically opaque. Strangest of all, while flesh was very transparent, bones were fairly opaque. And so the discoverer, interposing his hand between the source of the rays and his bit of luminescent cardboard, *saw* the bones of his living hand projected in silhouette upon the screen. The great discovery was made.[6]

Clearly, the X ray lent itself conveniently to the metaphors of blinding natural light and penetrating vision so often evoked in the "great man" approach to science history. The prehistory of this apocryphal moment is cast as a Miltonian narrative about "making darkness visible," a story in which these terms function both metaphorically and literally. The chief elements of this tale center on late-nineteenth-century physics and experiments in electricity, and the story unfolds as follows: Physicists observed the effects of currents produced in evacuated tubes containing an induction coil. The electromagnetic vibrations produced were observed through a glass window in the induction chamber. Desiring to observe the path of the electrons as they escaped from the tube, the Hungarian physicist Philipp Lenard substituted a thin aluminum sheet for the impervious glass window. The particles' passage through the aluminum screen was registered by a paper coated in a substance that would fluoresce on contact with the particles. In conducting such experiments, Lenard and other physicists noted that photographic film that happened to be in the room during this procedure often became fogged, despite a complete absence of light rays. But they were unable to explain this phenomenon and uninterested in pursuing it.

In November 1895, Roentgen reproduced Lenard's procedure with a different object in mind besides explaining this photographic effect. He set out to test the accepted idea that cathode rays did not penetrate glass. In the course of this experiment, he shielded the glass cover of a Crookes tube with a sheet of black cardboard impervious to cathode rays. He then noted, by chance, that a barium-platynocide-coated screen that happened to be lying nearby was fluorescing despite the complete blockage of the rays' passage out of the tube. He suspected that some other type of ray than cathode or light must be activating the screen.[7] He then devoted seven weeks to intensive study of what he supposed to be a new kind of ray.

Roentgen's report on this seven-week project contains an extensive account of his experimental procedure and empirical findings. He determined that the "mysterious rays" caused certain substances to fluoresce, were highly penetrating, exposed photographic plates, and resisted refraction, reflection, and deflection. His studies indicated that the entity causing the fluorescence was not light, cathode, or ultraviolet rays, but a hitherto unrecognized kind of radiation.[8] He could not, however, conclusively answer the question he posed in his report, "What, then, are these rays?" The generic designation "X rays," coined by Roentgen "for the sake of brevity," indicates the full extent of his knowledge of the mysterious entity's composition. Justifying the designation of the force he assumed to be behind the effects he perceived as rays, he cites the existence of the exposed photographic paper. The photograph thus stands as proof and justification of his identification of the mysterious force as a new kind of ray:

> The justification of the term "rays," applied to the phenomena, lies partly in the regular shadow pictures produced by the interposition of a more or less permeable body between the source and a photographic plate or fluorescent screen.[9]

The presence of an image bolstered what was in fact only a presumption that a new form of radiation has been discerned. An image registered on the photographic plate thus gained the status of experimental proof; the ray remained an undiscovered entity even after the appearance of its effects in the form of an image. Yet Roentgen's report was received in the popular and scientific press as a discovery of a new force in nature, and not of a new technique. The publication of Roentgen's report on his seven-week study quickly circulated, in the words of the Roentgen Ray Society president, "with telegraphic speed over the world," catapulting him to international fame as the "discoverer" of a still-unknown entity.

The technique that Roentgen introduced with his X-ray experiments was the subject of public hysteria not because it was shockingly new but because it ushered into the realm of science a disturbing technique of bodily representation long circulating in areas less invested than physics with epistemological authority—namely, popular metaphysics and public entertainment. For example, in the 1862 British stage illusion "Pepper's Ghost," conducted by civil engineer Henry Dirks and John Henry Pepper of the London Polytechnic Institute, mirrors and lights created the illusion of a man in a coffin dissolving into his skeleton.[10] This stage trick suggests a fascination with the illusionistic and metaphysical deployment of light as a force that may uncover truths about death and afterlife. The metaphysical-epistemological implications of this stage trick are that light no longer simply reflects off the surface of an object of knowledge, having shone upon it so that we may better observe it. Rather, light becomes a brutal force that physically penetrates its object, stripping away its concealing surface to lay its structure bare. It must have been with some consternation that the public saw this technique transformed from stage illusion to science. Indeed, at the time of Roentgen's report, this view of the body's susceptibility to light had already surfaced in medicine. At the turn of the century, lights were inserted in interior spaces like the bladder, the gastrointestinal tract, and the vagina to illuminate the tissue of organ walls from within much as a light bulb illuminates a lampshade. The physical and metaphorical power of penetrative light in these experiments was quite seductive, leading some physicians and scientists to make hasty claims about their heightened access to knowledge about the body. A 1903 issue of the *New York State Journal of Medicine* reports a physician's claim to have made "photographs taken by the light which had passed completely through the body of a stout man."[11] Examination of journals devoted to experiments in electricity shows that the use of light transillumination for imaging and diagnosis prefigures and parallels similar uses of the X ray, with an industry forming by midcentury around the production of various types of endoscopic devices and procedures based on this early technique.[12] Edison's comment that he would soon be able to photograph the brain through the skull provoked an enormous public response, including requests from readers to be the subject of these photographs (figure 5.1).[13] In the same year, a New York physician

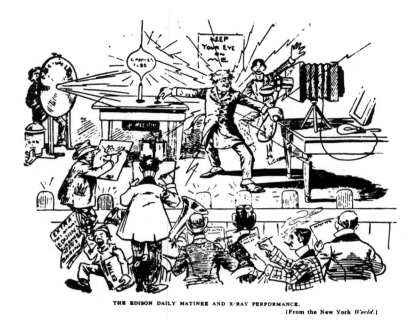

THE EDISON DAILY MATINEE AND X-RAY PERFORMANCE.
[From the New York *World*.]

Figure 5.1. Cartoon satirizing Edison's attempt to image the brain and capture an audience at the same time (*New York World,* 22 February 1896).

claimed that he had already used electric light rays in conjunction with sound to illuminate "the internal chamber of the brain."[14] Roentgen's "discovery" was received with such widespread excitement, then, because it further legitimated this model of visual knowledge as corporeal penetration and invasion, a model that previously had currency as popular fantasy and public spectacle.

The idea of the spectacle of the skeletal image of Roentgen's own living hand on the fluorescing screen, and the actual X-ray photograph of the hand of his wife, Bertha Roentgen, fascinated the medical profession and the lay public in 1896. Roentgen's rise to media stardom is somewhat ironic. In fact, his initial studies were conducted with the utmost secrecy. His biographer, Otto Glasser, speculates that this secrecy was prompted by the fact that the X-ray image of the skeleton immediately suggested itself to Roentgen as a cultural representation of death, and the physicist feared that his apparent foray into the realm of metaphysics would bring him disrepute among scientists:

> One can only imagine how this first ghostly shadow picture of the human skeleton within living tissue affected the observer. Doubt must have been followed by wonder, and perhaps by a reluctance to continue experiments that promised to

bring him disrepute in the eyes of his colleagues. At that point he determined to continue his experiments in secrecy.[15]

After viewing his own hand under the fluorescing screen, Roentgen subjected his wife's body to the same technique. But although he merely viewed his own hand under the fluoroscope in the privacy of his laboratory, he produced a photograph of his wife's hand, a reproducible image that could be circulated and reprinted in the scientific press (figure 5.2). This photograph, regarded as the earliest X-ray photograph of a human body, was widely published and bore an enormous symbolic weight in public culture. According to Glasser, the cultural meanings that the image would bear were not lost on Roentgen's wife:

> When [Roentgen] showed the picture to her, she could hardly believe that this bony hand was her own and shuddered at the thought that she was seeing her skeleton. To Mrs. Roentgen, as to many others later, this experience gave a vague premonition of death.[16]

Among the many physicians who immediately repeated Roentgen's experiments, a woman's hand, sometimes captioned as "a lady's hand," or "a living hand," became a popular test object. A particularly fine-boned appendage, the hand was a convenient entity because it could be imaged relatively easily (much like the frog and tadpole discussed in chapter 4). But hand X-ray images became popular items outside medical practice as well. The historian Stanley Reiser relates that "New York women of fashion had X-rays taken of their hands covered with jewelry, to illustrate that beauty is of the bone and not altogether of the flesh" (or, to use a more familiar turn of phrase, is not just skin deep), while married women gave X rays of their hands (presumably with wedding ring affixed, like Bertha Roentgen's hand) to their relatives.[17]

In the public sphere as in medicine, the female hand X ray became a fetish object par excellence. In an early discussion of fetishism, Freud refers to the practice of foot binding, wherein the foot is mutilated and then venerated.[18] Here, the hand is symbolically mutilated and then venerated as an icon of timeless feminine beauty. This image suggested that the female body, like the fetish object, is ownable (as the wedding band, visible in the X-ray image, seems to suggest). But, as Reiser's anecdote indicates, this fascination with the hand apparently was not limited to male viewers, as this photograph from 1896 demonstrates (figure 5.3).

The hand X ray also hinted at the possibility of an abhorrent apparition of a whole X-rayed body, flayed and bloodless. The image was received with both pleasurable fascination and dread, in part because the hand X ray froze in time a moment before the more significant threat posed in the spectacle of the whole-body X ray.[19] As a New York physician explained in 1896:

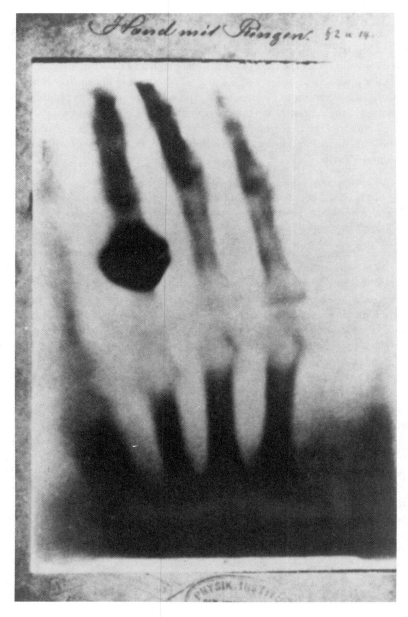

Figure 5.2. Bertha Roentgen's hand X ray, 1896.

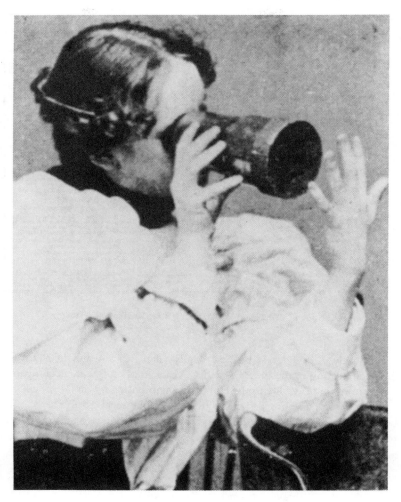

Figure 5.3. A woman using a fluoroscope to view her hand in X ray (photograph from 1896).

The surgical imagination can pleasurably lose itself in devising endless applications of this wonderful process. If it becomes possible to drive these mysterious rays through the entire body as clearly as they now penetrate the hand, the realm of utility will be practically boundless.[20]

As a highly charged site for the manifestation of anxieties about sexual difference, mutilation, and death, the spectacle of the X ray also provoked a riot of interpretive attacks and rejections. Although it was many years before a

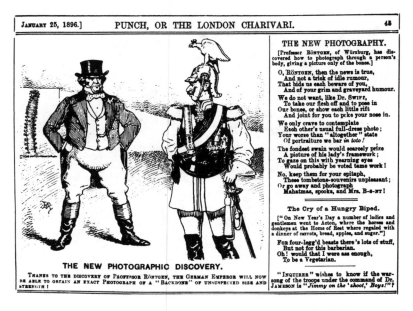

Figure 5.4. The poem "The New Photography"as it appeared in *Punch* (1896).

whole-body X ray would be successfully taken, the images of hands and limbs circulating in the press in the few years after 1896 were accompanied by cartoons that gave life to the fantasy of the monstrous whole-body X ray. The fascination and horror with which the public received the early X-ray body-part images is made quite explicit in the following two texts, the first a poem, "The New Photography," that appeared in *Punch* in 1896 (figure 5.4).

> *O, Röntgen, then the news is true*
> *And not a trick of idle rumour,*
> *That bids us each beware of you*
> *And of your grim and graveyard humour.*
>
> *We do not want, like Dr. Swift,*
> *To take our flesh off and to pose in*
> *Our bones, to show each little rift*
> *And joint for you to poke your nose in.*

We only crave to contemplate
Each other's usual full-dress photo,
Your worse than "altogether" state
Of portraiture we bar in toto!

The fondest swain would scarcely prize
A picture of his lady's framework;
To gaze on this with yearning eyes
Would probably be voted tame work!

No, keep them for your epitaph,
These tombstone-souvenirs unpleasant;
Or go away and photograph
Mahatmas, spooks, and Mrs. B-s-nt![21]

Expressed in this poem is a pervasive cultural anxiety over the X ray's perceived capacity to dissolve sexual identity by figuratively decomposing the organs and flesh. At stake is the loss of the cultural text inscribed in the skin, the organs. Clearly, for this author desire depends on the presence of a surface that conceals living structure, a signifying surface of clothing or skin that can be read for signs of sexual and cultural difference.[22] Hence, although the image of the concealing surface ("the full-dress photo") is "craved," a picture of structure itself ("his lady's framework") is "tame" stuff (figure 5.5).

Linda Williams has shown that in hard-core pornography it is not the actual sight of the genitals themselves but the ritual of concealment and unconcealment, and the narrative anticipation of visual revelation and climax, that is invested with erotic meaning.[23] The *Punch* poem seems to suggest that a similar logic was at work in the early regard of the X ray. Stripped of its flesh and other organs, the fully exposed skeleton was a boring sight. However, one might also conjecture that the author's apparent lack of interest is belied by his insistence that the X ray be censored ("we bar in toto"). While the abstract microscopic image of the fragmented, dissected body was received with responses ranging from indifference to wonder and aesthetic appreciation, the X ray, though also an abstraction and fragmentation of the body, was more frequently regarded as socially transgressive. The following editorial illustrates quite well this view of the X ray as a transgressive image.

We are sick of the Roentgen rays. . . . The consequence of which appears that you can see other people's bones with the naked eye. . . . On the revolting indecency of this there is no need to dwell. But what we seriously need to put before the government is that the moment tungstate of calcium [a substance marketed

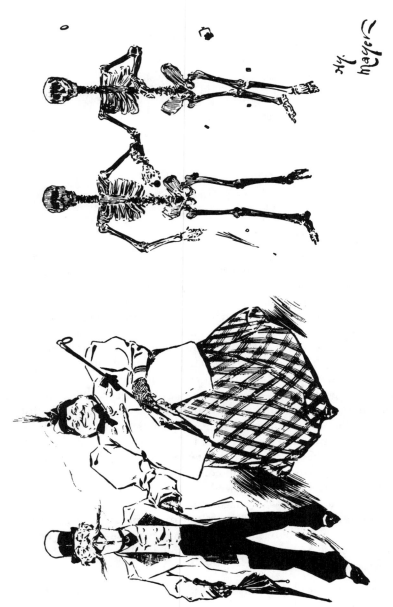

Figure 5.5. The caption to this cartoon from 1897 suggests that this cartoonist saw the X rays as a force that erased difference: "Whether stout or thin, the x-ray makes the whole world kin."

by Edison as an X-ray-sensitive medium] comes into anything like general use, it will call for legislative restriction of the severest kind. Perhaps the best thing would be for all civilized nations to combine to burn all works on the roentgen rays, to execute all the discoverers, and to corner all the tungstate in the world and whelm it in the middle of the ocean. Let the fish contemplate each other's bones, but not us.[24]

For this apopleptic author, the X ray signifies the ultimate violation of the boundaries that define subjectivity and identity, exposing the private interior to the gaze of medicine and the public at large. Indeed, the author regards this mode of seeing as so transgressive that it must be subject to "legislative restriction of the severest kind," its "discoverers" executed and its material evidence burned. This remarkably violent response suggests that the X-ray image was regarded as destructive both corporeally and morally. It is remarkable, though, that this passage does not draw for support on the medically documented cases of actual bodily decomposition and death caused by prolonged exposure to radiation. Instead, the author fixes on the supposed moral implications of exposing structure, a project that is ridiculed in the *Punch* poem but here rejected as a transgressive countercultural project, in keeping with pornography or spiritualism (the spiritualist's heretical revelation of the soul and his or her affinities with Eastern religions, for example).

In linking the X ray to these "uncivilized" practices, the authors of these texts are not far off the mark. Just before the 1896 X-ray mania, the British spiritualist and birth control activist/educator Annie Besant (the "Mrs. B–s–nt" our *Punch* author deems deserving of radiation exposure) brought out her book *The Self and Its Sheaths*, a title evoking an X-ray-like image of a stripping of the body's surface to its spiritual core. The X-ray photograph was in fact viewed by some spiritualists as an image of the soul, an association also made by many religious lay viewers not engaged in the subculture of spiritualism. Besant and "Mahatmas" (presumably meaning Indian religious leaders, a reference to the writers Besant appropriated in her spiritual writings) are sentenced to the X rays because they are viewed as embodying similarly marginal perspectives on social and political life and death.[25] In the popular press, cartoons abounded throughout the century featuring women stripped of their clothing by voyeuristic men wielding X-ray devices, as in this 1934 cartoon of *Ballyhoo*'s "candid X-ray cameraman" (figure 5.6). Glasser attributes popular and subcultural appropriations of the X ray to the lay public's ignorance. However, I would argue that the public showed great acuity in recognizing that the X ray was a radically new way of viewing and organizing the body, and in trying to appropriate it as such. It is perfectly true that the image of Bertha Roentgen's hand was in fact an object "gazed on with yearning eyes" not only by the popular press but by radiologists entranced by the stunning spectacle of death in life. And on another level, it

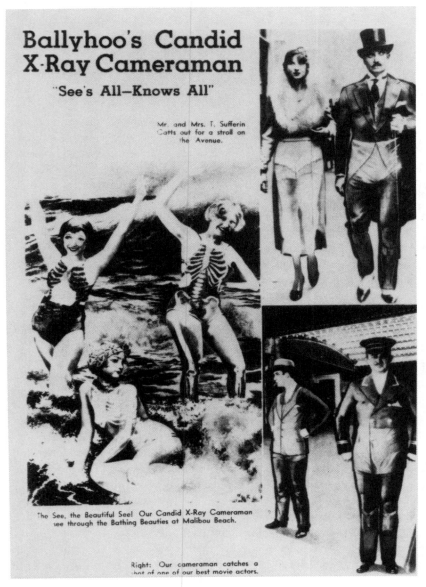

Figure 5.6. A 1934 cartoon reflecting popular fantasies about X-ray vision.

was more than clear that the penetrative gaze would effect dramatic changes in the medical treatment of bodies.

That the X ray was institutionalized in the first half of the century not only as a form of diagnosis but as a fetish object *and* as a powerful means of disciplining the body is clearly illustrated in Thomas Mann's 1927 novel *The Magic Mountain*. This narrative of sexualized death, which is set in a tuberculosis sanitarium, demonstrates the impossibility of considering medical techniques apart from their cultural meanings vis-à-vis life, sexuality, health, and death. In a particularly telling passage, the novel's protagonist, Hans Castorp, awaits his turn to be given a diagnostic X ray. He spies another patient, a young woman he admires and about whom he fantasizes in terms of a distinctively skeletal erotics. The description of his view of her body suggests an economy of desire organized around a body wasted not only by illness but by X rays:

> Chauchat had crossed one leg over the other again, and her knee, even the whole slender thigh, showed beneath the blue skirt. . . . She sat leaning forward, with her crossed forearms on her knee, her shoulders drooping, and her back rounded, so that the neck-bone stuck out prominently, and nearly the whole spine was marked out under the close-fitting sweater.[26]

The young man imagines himself in the place of the sanitarium's head doctor, Hofrat Behrens, who is also a painter for whom this woman models, in order to evoke an image of her skeletal body unclothed. This voyeuristic fantasy is abruptly checked, however, by the intrusive knowledge of the X-ray gaze, a technique also used by the doctor to image Chauchat—a technique whose very presence short-circuits the fantasy and elicits disavowal.

> Hans Castorp recalled, suddenly, that she too was sitting here waiting to be x-rayed. The Hofrat painted her, he reproduced her outward form with oil and colours upon the canvas. And now, in the twilighted room, he would direct upon her the rays which would reveal to him the inside of her body. When this idea occurred to Hans Castorp, he turned away his head and put on a primly detached air; a sort of seemly obscurantism presented itself as the only correct attitude in the presence of such a thought.[27]

The specter of the X ray catches Castorp in the act of looking, surprising him and disturbing his surreptitious fantasy by reminding him that, like Chauchat, he himself will soon be subject to the disciplining of a pervasive gaze that will symbolically waste away the flesh that his disease is already consuming. With this revelation, Castorp's identificatory affiliation abruptly shifts from the figure of the doctor to the object of his look. Finding himself caught in the field of the X ray with Chauchat, Castorp assumes "a primly detached air," feigning indifference as a defense against the specter of this woman's skeletal body and the threat it symbolizes regarding his own. Rendered speechless by this thought, his anxieties are succinctly articulated for him by the doctor: "I expect, Castorp, you feel a little nervous about exposing your inner self to our gaze?"[28]

Behrens tries to disengage Hans Castorp from his masochistic identifica-

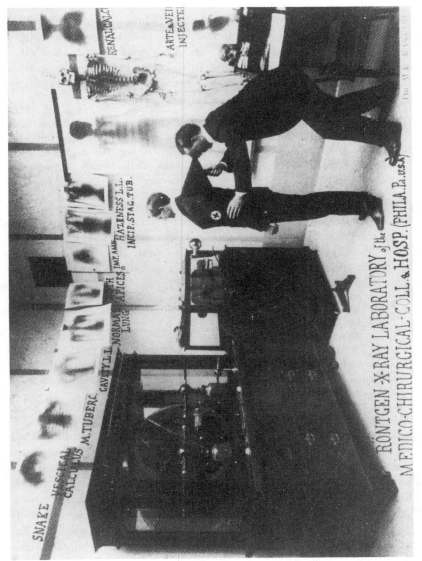

Figure 5.7. A turn-of-the-century X-ray clinic not unlike the one described in *The Magic Mountain*.

tion with the "feminine" state of being decomposed by disease and the X ray, encouraging him to enjoy the paradoxical spectacle of death that surrounds them in his X-ray-lined inner chamber (figure 5.7). Pointing to one of the skeletal images that line his laboratory walls, he explains, "There is the female arm, you can tell by its delicacy. That's what they put around you when they make love, you know."[29] But Castorp is unable to break his too-close identification with the image, or to elide the gaze. He again tries to distance himself by feigning indifference: "Very interesting," he flatly remarks of the doctor's macabre display. The potential thrill of looking is barred from his mind as he focuses instead on his own impending submission to the gaze.

In the following section, I consider in greater depth the responses of physicians and scientists like Dally who submitted their own bodies as test objects in their experiments with the X ray, giving up their lives in the process. I read these case histories of martyrs to the X ray in order to emphasize that the perverse spectatorial pleasure-in-looking represented in the figure of the doctor described above fully explains neither the cultural function of the X ray nor the subjectivity of its technician. It is impossible to view the physician or researcher only as voyeur or as sadistic agent of the gaze. As the case of Castorp begins to suggest, a much more complex and contradictory relation of identification and exposure exists among bodies, images, and cultural apparatus.

Throughout this book, I have attempted to analyze the ways that imaging technician and imaged subject are disciplined differently, and resist differently, within particular optical systems. I noted in the previous chapter that, although recent work on imaging techniques has emphasized technicians and their subjective acts of looking, much work in contemporary film theory has emphasized the spectator, a figure who, like the technician, is also a subject who looks. I have tried to pose the question of how the techniques I consider situate those living bodies who are placed on the scientific stage, subject to the scrutiny of a central authority, seen but not seeing. But what can be said of technicians who present their own bodies as chief objects of the scientific gaze? And what can one say about "seeing the body" when the very act of illuminating it destroys it? The discussion of the self-designated "martyrs to the X ray" that follows makes clear the impossibility of identifying the technician, scientist, or physician as the seat of authority in techniques of medical power. Rather, the technician of the gaze occupies an unstable position that at times merges with that of patient and object.

Martyrs to the X Ray

Patients' X-ray-induced conditions were not frequently the subject of the kind of professional documentation that we saw in the account of Edison's

X-ray illness. In the early documentation of experiments with the ray, we hear more often about miraculous cures and brilliant diagnoses. One explanation for this unbalanced reporting is that, as the report on Edison's symptoms suggests, the damaging effects of the rays often appeared years after experiments had first taken place. Because physical effects often appeared belatedly, reports on the association between X rays and cancer were often received by doctors and scientists with great skepticism. Another explanation, though, is that these professionals were trained to maintain a relationship of cool, objective distance from their "test objects"—even when these objects were living human beings. As we saw in the case of Bernard and others, the detachment with which many researchers regarded their living objects often escalated to sadistic mastery and detached indifference regarding the body's experience and fate. Yet, in the case of the Clarks, we also saw that the experiment can be a site for the investment of "family values" in the laboratory setting. Warmth, maternal nurturing, and community activity were incorporated into the production of new technological forms of life. In all of these cases, however, researchers went to great lengths to deny the evidence of correlation between technique and pain or death, focusing on signs of life even when its opposite was a seemingly indisputable fact.

Early experimentation on the X ray was no exception to this pattern, even when the test object in question was a person and the "experiment" took place in the course of medical treatment. For example, a New York physician relates a case of 1903 in which he subjected his patient to a twenty-minute X-ray exposure as experimental therapeutic treatment for a broken arm. Days after the X ray was administered, the patient developed a fever and blisters and swelling in the irradiated area. She died shortly thereafter. The physician initially considered as possible causes of death suicide, exhaustion, shock brought on by autosuggestion, and heart disease. Only after these causes were ruled out did he request an autopsy. He found that the woman's hip in the area "below the waist band, just where the X ray would strike the body unprotected by the elbow," had also become blistered, swollen, and infected. Further, her heart contained colonies of streptococcus, a sign of septicemia (blood poisoning). Though X-ray exposure had already been linked to septicemia, the physician refused to acknowledge the X ray as a possible cause of death.[30]

Denial in cases like this is difficult to understand, but more perplexing still are cases like that of Dally, described at the beginning of this chapter. The X-ray technician, whose body was continually close to the instrument, was more often the one to experience extreme pathological "side effects." A privileged viewer of some of the earliest radiographic representations, the technician was also among the earliest "test sites" for unplanned experiments on the effects of the rays. In 1896, an electrician named Elihu Thomson conducted one of the earliest documented tests on X-ray safety. Taking his own body as his test object, Thomson describes what must have been a quite painful experience of physical deterioration. I reproduce a lengthy passage from his report both to underscore the fact that detailed evidence of the X rays' pathological effects existed almost as soon as experiments with them began, and to provide an example of the clinical detachment with which many researchers regarded their own bodies:

> I was interested sometime ago in regard to the effect of Rontgen rays on tissues. I had read a few times that people had been burned by Rontgen rays. I did not believe it. These rays went through tissue so easily that their action could not amount to anything, but it was certainly worthwhile investigating so as to know. . . . I exposed the finger for half an hour to the rays. . . . I put the finger up pretty close to the tube, and after half an hour I thought that perhaps it was not long enough, perhaps it was not half long enough. But if there were to be any effect it would be equivalent to a few hours distance, and as I got tired I went no farther. I shut down the tube and went away. Five, six, seven, eight days passed and nothing happened, and I felt that people had been mistaken about the effect of the rays. But on the ninth day the finger began to redden; on the twelfth day there was a blister, and a very sore blister. On the thirteenth and fourteenth day after exposure, the blister had included all the skin down to the part not exposed and had gone around the finger almost to the other side. The whole of the epidermis came away and left an ulcer without any possibility of recovering its own epidermis except from the edges and I had to go through that painful process of having a raw sore there and the epidermis growing in from the side and gradually closing up. Only three days ago was the sore actually closed, and the skin is yet very tender, and nature does not appear to have found out how to make a good skin over that finger. The skin still comes off in flakes and is very disagreeable and very tender, and there is a burning, smarting, sensation every now and then. But I am satisfied that it is coming out all right. . . . This has taken six and a half weeks today.[31]

Surprisingly, Thomson's account did little to dissuade others from persisting with X-ray research. Reports that corroborated his findings were routinely challenged in professional circuits. Finally, what was at stake in these debates was not causality at all. Even in the face of incontestable proof that the rays could cause such things as dermatitis, blindness, arthritis, blood poisoning, leukemia, and cancer, physicians and researchers persisted in their experiments. Denial of the rays' potential pathological effects was replaced by an embrace of these effects in the name of a greater good.

The autobiography of the physician, radiologist, and industrialist Emil Grubbé demonstrates this response.[32] In a chapter devoted to "the effects of the X-rays on the author's body," Grubbé coolly outlines in detail the gradual deterioration of his flesh as he subjected his body to X-ray testing. He describes his gradual loss of body parts, beginning with his fingers "a joint or two at a time . . . by this slow-death process." The clinical objectivity with

which he relates his bodily decomposition to the reader replicates his laboratory method: in order to analyze more closely the effects of X rays on tissue,
he sliced minute bits from his amputated joints and viewed them under the
microscope. This penchant for distanced analysis and self-mutilation, however, leaves off with Grubbé's account of his social life. He describes the
painful experience of being unable to shake hands with his one intact but ulcerated hand, an appendage whose "wrinkled, shriveled, and lifeless" form
deeply embarrassed him. Ironically, the very appendage whose X-ray image
had come to symbolize eternal life and beauty was here identified as
grotesque and deathly. No longer able to maintain his thriving business of
manufacturing X-ray equipment, Grubbé devoted what remained of his life
to the practice and teaching of the science of X rays, though this work too
was hampered by his inability to enunciate (his cancerous upper lip having
been removed). "For fear of not being understood," he concluded, "I would
rather not speak at all."

Grubbé not only accepted these multiple forms of mutilation and this
"slow-death process," he masochistically embraced them. Through subjection to the rays, he was exalted (in his own words) as the "founder" of X-ray
therapy, and as a sovereignly chosen subject of scientific knowledge. "It was
evident," he stated, "that my body had been made a testing laboratory."[33]
He reveals in the following passage exactly who chose him for this job:

> Nature assigned this job to me, and I consider it a privilege to have done the job
> which was allotted to me. I have lived to see the child that I fathered develop
> into a sturdy, mature and worthwhile product; and I hope, as I approach the
> evening of my day, to see even more uses for x-ray therapy in the alleviation of
> the ills of mankind.[34]

This is truly a peculiar twist: nature makes a human body a laboratory, with
its instruments, equipment, and technology. Grubbé's account is an extreme
example of the submission of the technician and his "natural" body to the
"death ray" and its powerful technological apparatus. His story is instructive,
though, because it makes clear a problem in theorizing agency: it becomes
difficult to analyze the distinction among subjects, objects, and agency in the
cultural apparatus of radiography. Radiographic knowledge (information
about dosage, image interpretation and use, and so on) is acquired only at the
expense of test bodies. Because of his proximity to the instrument, the radiographer was often the person whose body was given up to the process, will-
ingly or not. As I have noted elsewhere in this book, the tendency in the
analysis of scientific knowledge has been to think the observer as one who
remains psychically removed from the experimental object. And in the
analysis of the cinema, the tendency has been to think the observer as one
who remains physically distanced from the profilmic object. But here the
subject looking is quite literally caught and punished by the surveillant appa-

ratus whose rays do not restrict themselves to the intended object but range out to incorporate the technician. Yet, though he is punished for his act of looking, the radiographer is also rewarded for giving himself up to a greater public good. For his bodily submission, he is offered an exalted place in an afterlife where the individual subject may still hold a privileged place of authority—in the history of medicine. The debasement and masochism inherent in the role of the technician who gets too close with his machine and who confuses himself with his object are thus managed by another cultural apparatus, the writing of medical history as a narrative of great men and their selfless devotion to research.

As the X ray became a more pervasive technique of medical diagnosis and therapy, this issue of X-ray dosage became more urgent. In order to determine what constituted a dangerous exposure, however, radiologists first needed to be able to measure and compare the exposures they administered, and then regulate that dosage. This was no easy task. Different equipment generated different amounts of radiation, and without a standard means of measuring radiation it was impossible to compare data. Furthermore, there was no clear idea about what exactly should be measured, since the process included factors such as object density, distance of object from the apparatus, and duration of exposure. All of these factors varied widely within and among practices. There was also a perceived need to standardize techniques for producing and reading X-ray images. Though standardization of dosage and image quality is still a crucial part of maintaining safe and effective X-ray practice, it continues to be an impossibly complex issue (as I will show in the next chapter).

Some of the problems in establishing quantitative standards are suggested in an account from 1913 by a physician frustrated with the lack of correlation among different X rays of a single case. He suggests that standardization might be possible if "all radiographs in a case [be] taken by one man." This idea implies that the image itself is a less reliable indicator than the subjective procedure of the individual technician. In other words, the activity of the technician himself is more consistent than the subjective, even capricious, tendencies of the group and its various instruments.[35] This idea is a peculiar reversal of the logic of the astronomical observatory described by Shaffer, a process in which human observation was regarded as subjective and subject to corrective instrumentation. But it is contradicted in a report on dosimetry published a decade later, which is devoted almost entirely to the difficulties of establishing a technical norm. The author notes that the energy transported in the X ray is so small that it is nearly indiscernible; variables such as apparatus used, absorption of rays by surrounding surfaces (variations in tissue density and composition), wavelength of radiation, and frequency of exposure made it difficult to forecast actual exposure even with a set standard in place. Echoing Arago's suggestion that the photosensitive surface could be used to document light intensity itself, the author suggests that photographic film (rather than a human manager) would be the most accurate register of dosage.[36]

Dosage measurement was an especially crucial science for researchers trying to combine the techniques of film and X ray. The many images required for even a short strip of film and the brevity of each image's exposure demanded that a very high cumulative level of radiation be used to expose even a short strip of film. The inability to regulate exposure conditions adequately made motion-picture X rays of human subjects a dangerous prospect. As Michaelis summed up the problem at midcentury, "the most powerful source of X-rays is the essential requirement for cinematography. This requirement is in conflict with the safety of the patient.[37] If the thrill of danger accompanied X-ray experiments, X-ray cinematography posed the ultimate thrill. As we shall see, the threat of radiation was the price paid for reinvesting the deathly, bloodless X-ray body with the signifiers of life. The X-ray cinema imbued the pathological image with a hyperreal semblance of movement, depth, blood, and flesh. As we shall see, the X-ray image is even given a voice.

When the Fetish Comes to Life: X-Ray Motion Pictures

Almost every historical account of X-ray cinematography begins by recounting John Macintyre's 1897 screening of motion picture X-ray footage of a frog's leg described in chapter 1.[38] Like Krogh and countless other laboratory researchers, he chose the frog because it was conveniently flat, thin skinned, and anatomically simple, and hence easily imaged with relatively low exposures. Macintyre subjected the frog to electrical stimulation and made a series of photographic plates of its leg movements. These were combined to make a short animated filmstrip, which he spliced into a loop for continuous projection.

Although Macintyre conducted his experiment in the laboratory, he clearly regarded his film as a source of popular amusement. He chose to demonstrate it for the first time not to a professional audience but to a group of professional and lay viewers gathered on Ladies' Night at the Glasgow Royal Society. Like Duchenne, whose microscopic lantern slides of histologic sections, as Gilman tells us, doubled as dinner party amusements, Macintyre's frog-leg film functioned both as popular spectacle and object of close analysis. Ladies' Night, like the dinner party, suggests an audience of women and men, scientists and lay viewers, and a scientist masquerading as entertainer, his presence authorizing this transposition of cultural forms. The scene evokes the genre of the animated cartoon, with its anthropomorphic animals and its spectacles of bodily contortion and fragmentation, as well as the anthropomorphizing, fragmenting, and contorting views of the scientific motion analysis. The similarity of these modes was not lost on the radiologist and filmmaker James Sibley Watson Jr., whose oeuvre includes a reel of cinematic animal X-ray experiments humorously titled "Disney Animal Review" (I will be returning to Watson's work shortly). When reprinted in professional journals and analyzed in the laboratory, these same films were cast as research material, ostensibly incomprehensible and off limits to the lay viewer, accessible only to an audience of trained observers.

Whereas the static X-ray photograph functioned as icon and fetish, a frozen moment of death in life, the moving X-ray image presented a different kind of spectacle—a spectacle of movement, and hence a more suitably physiological image. Macintyre's film was essentially a series of static photographs spliced together and projected. In 1910 a New York radiologist took tracings from X rays of gastric movements, photographing his drawings in succession to make an animated film.[39] But this technique could not display the actual rate of gastric movement. It is useful here to recall the case of Watkins, the physician who wanted to capture living blood flow on the microscope's stage. X-ray cinematography seemed to offer the possibility of seeing interior human physiology in living motion. But the factor of dosage interfered, threatening to destroy its object in the process of imaging it. A high cumulative dosage had to be used to expose the many frames composing the filmstrip. And, as was noted earlier in this chapter, higher dosage was also necessary to make an image of body parts other than bone. Thus, although it was possible to display animal skeletal activity in moving X rays (as Macintyre did), it was much more difficult to display the living movement of other physiological systems (the respiratory, circulatory, or digestive systems, for example), and nearly impossible to image the human body without the risk of damage. Nevertheless, the X-ray photograph was received by its viewers as a static and bloodless image evoking death, whereas the moving X ray suggested the potential to breath life into that image, animating it and investing it with newly configured surfaces and fluids, symbolic flesh and blood.

Radiological contrast media were key to this symbolic reconstitution of the body's flesh and blood. In part through the work of the well-known U.S. physiologist Walter Cannon (who died of an X-ray-induced blood disorder), it was found that X-ray-impervious substances such as barium or bismuth could be used to coat organs and passageways that didn't image well with X rays. Radiologists found that by feeding or injecting a substance that blocks X rays (a radiologically opaque, or radiopaque, substance) into the veins or the respiratory or digestive systems, for example, those processes that had previously been invisible under the rays were cast in relief. What was displayed, of course, was not the organ or passageway itself, but the opaque fluid coating its surfaces. By "painting" the permeable interior walls of organs with radiopaque media, much as one might paint a glass window to block out light, radiographers essentially implanted impenetrable surfaces where previously they had been erased by the rays. And by infusing a fluid contrast medium into passageways that carried gases (the respiratory system), radiographers in effect infused the static, bloodless X-ray image with life.[40]

The symbolic weight borne by the image of flow is well illustrated in the following X-ray experiment conducted in the late 1940s. A team of cardiologists at the University of Rochester devised a method for studying congenital heart defects with motion picture X rays. Their object of study was the newborn infant. In one of the short film studies produced by this team, the torso of an infant is shot in close-up. We see the blood, made visible with the injection of a contrast medium, coursing through its system in a short sequence representing eight real-time heartbeats. Projected in a continuous loop, these eight beats were viewed over and over, simulating the repetitive cycle of the blood. The idea behind this project was the discernment of congenital heart defects unable to be perceived by other means. There is no documentation on the success of the technique. However, my concern is not with the technique's viability or lack thereof, but with the cultural implications of this kind of optical investigation. One can find numerous instances in the study of human physiology in which the display of the flow of blood takes on a highly symbolic function.[41] But among the photographic and cinematic displays and analyses of living systems considered in this book, this experiment in infant cardiology most clearly exemplifies the deep scientific fascination with the image of life as a durational system—the "arrangement" of the living being that Bernard referred to in his account of his "experiments of destruction" described in chapter 2. In the films of infant angiography, on display is not only the flow of "life," but the observer's compulsion to display, reveal, and analyze bodies, and thereby vivify science. I would suggest that although the identification of pathology may very well have been the aim of the project, it is impossible to overlook its participants' fascination with viewing "new" life (a fascination that would soon feed the development of a thriving industry around obstetrical ultrasound), through a technique so strongly associated with the cultural iconography of death. Furthermore, the decision to loop-project the eight heartbeats represented in this film demands consideration in terms of the anxieties and pleasures associated with repetitive viewing.

Interestingly, Freud wrote about repetition compulsion in conjunction with the concept of birth trauma. While the essay hardly provides an adequate theoretical framework for analysis here, it can be usefully regarded as a symptomatic text with certain parallels to the case at hand. Freud had legitimate criticisms of Otto Rank's use of the concept of birth trauma, but he tacitly retained it as a prototype of sorts (rather than an origin) of "internal dangers," the experience of attack on the ego from within as a result of traumatic experience remaining as a "foreign" body "within" the subject.[42] It is worth noting that he took as a metaphor for this specter of a danger from within (and the desire to eliminate it) a trauma experienced by the fetal body in its passage out of the maternal body. However, a more apt model than the fetus for the situation he described is the figure of the pregnant woman, for whom the fetus might be said to be a "danger within." Freud described repetition compulsion in this context as the fixating factor in repression, the compulsion following the course of the repressed instinct "as though the successfully surmounted danger situation were still in existence."[43] One of three overdetermining factors he cited in the ego's struggle to undo its repressions is biological. He speculated that the protracted motor helplessness of the human infant is due to its too-brief intrauterine existence. Compared to other (unspecified) animals, the human infant, he explained, emerges relatively early, in an "unfinished" state. This biological circumstance is one factor predisposing the human being to a later experience of helplessness in the face of overwhelming automatic anxieties and a desire for a return to unity with the body of the mother.

Again, I do not bring up the concept of birth trauma here in order to revive it as an analytical model. However, I do want to suggest that this account displaces the site of trauma from maternal to fetal body, making the fetus available to the viewer as an identificatory figure. The X-ray studies of newborns described above perform a similar function, displacing anxiety about the traumatic sight of the maternal body in the process of birth to the body of the neonate. The radiographer obsessively searches and re-searches the same few frames of some of the newborn's earliest independent heartbeats for evidence of congenital damage, a heart defect noticeable only for a brief moment during the heart's movements and, until that moment, hidden away inside the maternal body. Here the infant, barely having emerged from that body (and, in Freud's view, still an "unfinished" project), is injected with a medium that might reveal an otherwise imperceptible "danger within."

The intentions of the physicians in their quest for signs of congenital pathology are not in dispute here. I do, however, want to highlight the peculiar displacement of anxieties about interiority and pathology, and the compulsive, repetitive act of their inquiry. The filmstrip is watched again and again for signs of pathology, as though with each revolution of the cycle the source of danger might suddenly reveal itself in the apparently normal image. This process recalls the peculiar microscopic experiments of Watkins—his attempts to coax out the "presymptom of the symptom," to make the body reveal signs of pathology to him even before the patient is aware of pathology's presence.

A striking precedent to these studies in infant angiography is a 1932 film of the respiratory system made by the German radiologist Robert Janker, a well-known researcher in radiology whose work was closely followed by the Rochester radiology team. The Janker film that I will shortly describe illustrates more clearly the complex ways that the moving X ray's "revolutionary" exposition of life and pathology is also linked to a fascination with death. Janker used visual repetition, movement, solidity, and depth to an unprecedented and ultimately lethal degree to reveal the living respiratory process.

Janker was one of a group of radiologists whose work became well known under the Nazi regime. From 1928 to 1937 he was director of the Roentgen Institute of the Bonn University Surgical Clinic, after which he established his own Roentgen Institute in Bonn. The short 1932 radiographic motion study that concerns me is included in a longer historical film recounting Janker's work to 1962. A print of this film was owned by the Rochester radiology department, and so would have been familiar to them.[44] The film in question records the passage of contrast medium from the trachea to the bronchi in a living cat. The cat is framed in a way that suggests that it is suspended or propped up (a vertical pose more common in humans than in animals). With each breath the cat takes, we see the contrast medium inhaled further into the bronchial tree. Over the course of less than a minute, every last branch fills in, becoming sharply delineated in the image. At the moment that the bronchi are fully engorged with contrast medium, Janker's voiceover narration (dubbed onto the film around 1962) concludes, "at last, even the finest bronchi can be seen" (figure 5.8). As the contrast fluid progressively fills the passageway, the cat's rate of respiration noticeably increases. What the voice-over does not mention is that this process is leading, as in Krogh's frog film, to the cat's death. Its quickening rate of respiration is a disturbing register of its struggle to breathe as the advancing fluid cuts off its air supply.

Here dimensionality, movement, and distinctions of object and ground—familiar conventions of a certain kind of pictorial realism—are critically tied to the animation of the death process. At the start of the film, the torso of the cat is in static profile, the passage of contrast medium the only movement in the shot. Its movement is two-dimensional and lateral to the focal plane. As the bronchial tree becomes nearly full, there is a match cut to a shot in which the torso of the cat is rotated on its axis—in other words, as the cat is about to die, its body is set in motion. The revolution of the cat's body imputes volume to the image, making the bronchial tree that is now so sharply delineated also suddenly fully dimensional. Janker's voice-over underscores the conventional realism of this shot: "The movement gives a three-dimensional impression."

Axial movement creates a stunning impact in the film partly because it heightens the illusion of dimensionality, but also because it turns the continuous flow of contrast medium into a repetitive cycle that introduces a greater

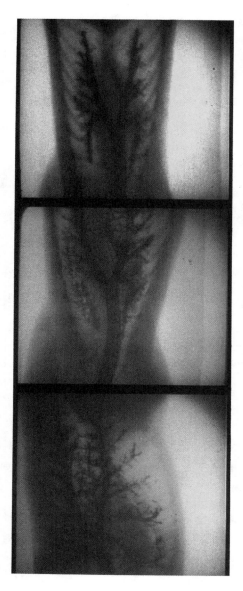

Figure 5.8. Frames from Janker's
motion study of a cat's bronchi.

degree of solidity and spatiality with each turn. As the cat's torso rotates, we
see the bronchi's "negative" space—the space previously filled with air—
more sharply in relief, more filled with contrast medium, more suffocatingly
real. Whereas earlier X-ray images described were markedly flat and static
(the timeless, flat image of the skeletal hand, for instance), here the death-

image is also a depth-image. In this film, familiar conventions of pictorial realism—depth, movement, object-ground correspondence—are linked to a distanced, sadistic gaze. Finally, Janker loses interest in the cat at the moment it ceases to breathe, and the film ends.

Drawing from Janker's method, the Rochester angiography films were remarkable for their time, not only because they made it possible to see subtle, momentary signs of human pathology that had been indiscernible, but because they depicted human torsos at a time when whole-body X-ray motion pictures were regarded as risky and off limits in most laboratories outside Germany (where X-ray investigations were conducted during the period with a stunning disregard for the safety of the imaged subject). It is important to note here that the films of Janker and the Rochester team were not shot directly in X ray but were filmed from the fluoroscopic screen. The fluoroscopic screen was introduced to the market by Edison and other early industrialists, and consisted of a screen coated with an X-ray-sensitive substance on which one could register in actual time the radiographic appearance of the moving body. It was used in locations ranging from the hospital (to perform routine chest X rays, discussed in the next chapter) to the shoe store (where it was a podiatric gimmick used ostensibly to determine the skeletal soundness of the customer's foot). By filming the real-time movement that appeared on the fluoroscopic screen, physicians could observe the moving scene afterward, without having to be present in the room while the X rays were being generated. The two projects I have just described were produced in this manner, eliminating the need directly to expose each film frame with X rays. Though image quality was diminished (this being essentially a form of rephotography), radiation levels were comparatively lower (though they would not qualify as "safe" by current standards).

A full discussion of the important issue of dosage levels and standardization would be too complex to include here. It is worth a brief digression, though, to note that the experiments in infant angiography were preceded by work with animals in the late 1920s through the early 1940s. These experiments were led by Stafford Warren, chief of the radiology department at Rochester's Strong Memorial Hospital. Warren, who in 1943 left Rochester to become the chief medical advisor for the Manhattan Project, was responsible for devising experiments for testing plutonium tolerance on human subjects. He led an experiment in which eleven Rochester patients were injected with forty times the amount of plutonium an average person could expect in a lifetime. The subjects were not informed of their role in this experiment, which was being conducted to test human tolerance of the strongly carcinogenic plutonium 239, one of the most toxic substances known, and one of the main ingredients in an atomic bomb. Scientists of the period believed that the dosages they administered were five and one-half times what a plutonium worker building atomic weapons would ingest over fifty years. Warren's role in this project might give some indication of his possible stance on concern about X-ray dosage versus the potential for scientific knowledge.[45] It is not surprising that this same figure was responsible for early X-ray experiments.

The fluoroscopic screen facilitated a return to a spectacle of human movement previously off limits to radiographers. The two films I have described are relatively early examples of the tendency to the spectacular that marks X-ray cinematography. Thus far, my discussion of the moving X ray has emphasized the reinvestment of those pictorial elements so carefully stripped from the scientific image in other contexts: depth of field, object-ground distinctions, perspectival space. But the animation of the death image also included techniques that ultimately cast the X-ray image squarely in the realm of popular spectacle. Whereas Macintyre's 1897 X-ray film functioned ambiguously as popular novelty and motion study research text, the moving X rays of the 1930s, 1940s, and 1950s were often quite unambiguously encoded as spectacle even in the scientific context.

In order to understand radiology's apparent move away from distanced, analytical viewing and toward "unscientific" spectatorial positions blatantly marked by pleasure, desire, voyeurism, or identification, it is necessary to return to a theme pursued in the previous chapter: the idea that scientific representational conventions are not distinct from those found in cultural movements associated with modernism, and that these separate institutions and contexts share techniques for disciplining, organizing, and generating life. In the concluding section of this chapter, I take as my case in point the oeuvre of James Sibley Watson Jr., a filmmaker and radiographer whose work engages this seemingly odd juxtaposition of interests.

A Physiological Modernism: X-Ray Cinema's Spectacle of Life

Watson was a participant in the team that produced the infant angiography project described above; he was also a part of the collaborative team that produced a definitive work of early U.S. film modernism, *The Fall of the House of Usher* (1929). More than twenty years before his work in X-ray cinema, Watson received an M.D. from New York University. However, he put aside medicine for a career in publishing. As editor during the 1920s of the magazine *The Dial* and as chief benefactor and intellectual supporter of such artists and writers as Gaston Lachaise, e. e. cummings, Marianne Moore, and Kenneth Burke, Watson established himself as a primary shaper of U.S. literary modernism. In 1929, he and the art historian and poet Melville Webber completed *The Fall of the House of Usher*, a short experimental adaptation of Edgar Allan Poe's story of the same title. With the completion of this film, Watson gave up his job at *The Dial* and focused more intensively on film production, collaborating with Webber on other experimental film projects, including the 1933 *Lot in Sodom*, a sound film loosely based on the biblical tale from Genesis—a film in which gay male desire figures strongly.[46] Watson thus established himself as a major figure in the early history of both literary and film modernism. During World War II, however, he resumed his medical career, initially specializing in the study of the gastrointestinal system. He is credited with the production of some of the first color photographs of the stomach's interior.[47] He joined the team of radiologists at Rochester in the mid-1940s, functioning as a central creative and technical source for a prolific X-ray motion picture practice that would extend into the 1960s.

Why this apparent break with avant-garde film aesthetics in favor of the clinical photography of the body's interior? A brief account of *The Fall of the House of Usher* may clarify the connection between these apparently disparate areas of film work. Poe's story centers on the characters of Madeleine and Roderick Usher, siblings (described as the last of their line) who occupy a crumbling family mansion, and a childhood friend of Roderick's who visits the home. The story's plot is minimal: Madeleine falls into a catatonic state and her brother temporarily entombs her in a vault in the cellar of the house, ostensibly to keep her body from the hands of certain "obtrusive" medical men eager to investigate her body for clues to the cause of her affliction. At the story's end, Madeleine rises up from her "region of horror" to "bear [her brother] to the ground a corpse."[48] Framed by brief shots of the visitor entering and leaving the Usher mansion, the fifteen-minute film takes place almost exclusively within the interior space of the house, a space that is encoded to resemble the interior space of a body. The film set evokes a painting described in the Poe story, a small picture rendered by Roderick and "representing the interior of an immensely long, rectangular vault or tunnel with low, smooth walls"—and a space that is apparently in the minds of Watson and Webber when they draw from the conventions of cubism to render the mansion's organic interior in a series of overlapping, graphically reduced, planar walls and surfaces. Following Madeleine's triumphant felling of her brother, the film closes with a highly abstract, graphic image of two torsolike figures—an image that strongly resembles an X ray of two bodies in its tonality, density, and composition.

This organization of the body is pervasive, extending beyond the techniques of modernist art and science. Artworks like Marcel Duchamp's *Nude Descending a Staircase*, Umberto Boccioni's X-ray-inspired pieces, or the time-lapse films of avant-garde filmmaker Germaine Dulac can easily be summoned to prove a thesis of the mutual influence of art and science. However, my point is that these works cannot be properly understood without reference to both the less canonical visual texts in laboratory science and medicine and the public responses to and influences on these images. Science and elite art are not impervious to cultural interpretations of each other's rar-

efied texts; as we saw earlier in this chapter, popular and subcultural knowledges of the body play a critical role in the development of these specialized
scientific and artistic techniques. To examine the cultural interpretations that
subtend Watson's work in avant-garde literature and film, I will now turn to
his popular science spectacles.

The Rochester team was not unique in its work on X-ray film motion
study. Significant work was done at the University of Toronto and at a range
of sites in the United States during the 1950s. However, I will continue to
focus on this group's work because it is one of the more prolific and lengthy
forays into the medical, scientific, and popular uses of moving X rays. The
infant angiography films were followed by numerous studies of animal and
human physiology, many of which were markedly ambiguous in their audience address. For example, the reel jokingly labeled "Disney Animal Review" includes footage of a live snake slinking along, a study requested by
scientists at Columbia University interested in proving a theory about the
mechanics of the snake's skeletal system. Among the Rochester team's numerous studies in physiology is footage of a curator of the George Eastman
House film collection guzzling an entire mug of beer in one gulp. This feat
is recorded as a scientific study in the mechanics of swallowing, though it
clearly also served as a source of amusement. In footage that will be discussed
at greater length in the next chapter, a scientific demonstration of the uses of
contrast media also comments on sexual difference and its relationship to visibility: gazing into a mirror, a man shaves away his image by using a razor to
remove contrast medium "shaving cream." A woman also stands before a
mirror, but her task is to apply contrast medium "makeup" in a process that
renders her face fully visible in X ray. In another reel, a woman gazes into a
compact as she applies lipstick, her image gradually dissolving into an X ray.
In this case, the X ray preserves rather than strips away signs of sexual difference (in the form of her feminine accoutrements—the compact and lipstick
tube) along with her bones (figure 5.9).

The Rochester team reproduced many of the moving X-ray "experiments" displayed in the numerous films of Janker and his colleagues, which
were available in their own collection and in the nearby Eastman House collection (a body of films that would also have been familiar to Watson
through his connections to the Rochester film and art community). We find
in the Rochester collection footage in which subjects comb their hair (the
metal comb visible in X ray), play musical instruments on sound film, and
perform all manner of everyday activity. These films recall the experiments
in human physiology conducted by Muybridge, mentioned in chapter 2
with reference to Linda Williams's analysis of them. As was noted earlier,
Williams points out that many of these ostensibly "purely scientific" images
are staged with a narrative and props, rendering them texts that function to
affirm and scientifically legitimate constructions of sexual difference. The

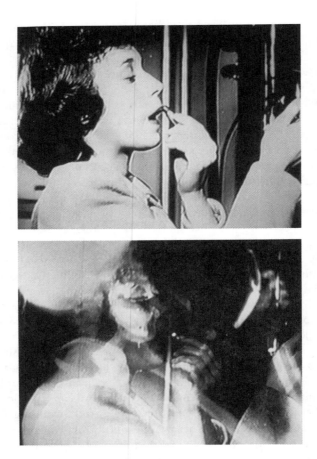

Figure 5.9. Frames from Paramount's *The Inside Story* (circa 1955)

Rochester films supplement this technique by reinvesting the X ray, an image that reveals human physiology at its modernist core, with the attributes of three-dimensionality and voice. As I have already shown, the body stripped of its signifying surface to reveal its "dead" structural bones is technologically invested with organs and "blood" that can be brought to life only by the X ray. The Rochester team takes this project of implanting life in the body to its mannerist limit, imputing a hyperreal dimensionality to the torso; sync-sound to that emblematic organ of life, the heart; and a proclivity for high culture to the vocal cords, which we see performing classical music in X ray.

In 1953, Watson and his colleagues announced the success of a new process for the production of three-dimensional motion picture X rays.

Janker had shown stereoscopic film heart studies at the 1937 German Congress of Radiology,[49] and Watson had access to prints of this work. A brief consideration of the meaning of the dimensional X-ray body in the German context is worth outlining. As background to the understanding of spatiality in German radiography, I refer to Robert Proctor's history of Nazi science. Although Proctor's book does not take on popular medical visual culture to any extent, his analysis touches interestingly on the cultural meanings of the full, corporeal body put forth in 3-D X-ray cinema, and their implication for the modernist culture of the flat described in the previous chapter. He cites one of the attempts by Nazi science to discredit the achievements of Jewish physicians and scientists:

> In 1936, Dr. Heinrich Chantraine published an article in the official journal of the Nazi Physicians' League claiming that Jews have problems with spatial and depth perception; this was why "the Jews never developed X-ray stereoscopy, even though they dominate the science of radiology."[50]

Proctor goes on to describe Chantraine's characterization of Jewish doctors and scientists as "technical" thinkers unable to grasp the fact that science springs from a "natural bond to nature." Interestingly, for Chantraine, technical thinking and the break with theories of the organic and nature are fundamentally linked to the aesthetic or conventions of flatness associated with modern art movements. Jewish art was always "two-dimensional," he stated; only Nordic man could see and build in three dimensions. Here the utopian form of the modernist aesthetic described in the previous chapter emerges as a break with racist science and its organization of the body as a full, completely spatialized real.

German radiography was not the only inspiration for the Rochester 3-D films. In the United States during the 1950s, there was a marked interest in expanding screen space in the popular cinema. In addition to screen-widening techniques such as CinemaScope, the industry introduced 3-D processes for imputing depth to the screen image. 3-D films became quite the rage in 1953 with the introduction of the first Cinerama feature, *This Is Cinerama*, which includes a harrowing roller coaster sequence. Most 3-D commercial releases featured perversions of nature (*Creature from the Black Lagoon*), often in the form of science fictions about outer space (*It Came from Outer Space*).[51] Although Watson and his colleagues were aware of Janker's earlier work, their project was clearly influenced by this 3-D craze in the United States, their fascination with inner space the flip side of the popular 3-D cinema's fascination with uncharted outer space.[52]

Janker (in the 1930s) and Watson after him (in the 1950s) augmented the 3-D view of the heart with synchronous soundtracks of the heartbeat. Like Janker's 1932 cat respiration study, in these films Watson's dimensional heart rotates on its axis, but now we may hear as well as see evidence of its living action. Recalling the cinematographic/kymographic apparatus of François-Franck, Janker further compounded this setup by reprinting an image of a kymographic record of the heart, taken simultaneously with the cinefluorographic study, along the edge of the image field. The two discrete records of living action are thus joined in one image, just as the sound and image tracks are "married" in the visual encoding of the optical soundtrack on the edge of the filmstrip. Thus a synchronous "real-time" record of image, sound, and graphic inscription accrues in the moving image—a veritable barrage of technologies for the surveillance of life.[53] The horrific threat of the X ray, posed both in its actual threat of decomposition and death and its metaphorical reference to the afterlife, seems to have given rise to a radiological frenzy to cover over the death image, reinscribing it with layer upon layer of signifiers of life. The stereoscopic, sync-sound, kymographic moving X ray is finally the overinvested site of a massive historical denial.

Throughout this chapter I have spoken of the X ray as a charged site of cultural meanings, but I have not always been specific about the nature of those meanings in terms of subjects and their cultural identities. I will conclude this chapter with a brief consideration of the nationalistic implications of Janker's work. In one of his sync-sound cinefluorographic records of human physiology, Janker films the larynx during speech. The voice he records is a male voice, a man delivering a nationalist speech. This film was produced during the Third Reich, and was clearly viewed as a timely opportunity to inscribe the full, living radiographic body as an emblem of national identity. X-ray technology in Germany in the 1930s and 1940s was advanced on the backs of citizens subjected to dosages that most certainly caused serious health problems later in life. Not all of these subjects were aware of their status as sacrificial object, and (as, for example, in the case of enforced sterilization by X ray) not all participants in radiological experiments understood the force of the medium. The film in question displays a subject whose image is marked in advance with the signs of his own eventual decomposition and death through imaging. Like Edison's deaf-mute girl who "sings" "The Star-Spangled Banner," this X-ray body speaks a nationalist text. Just as the turn-of-the-century film fails to transform the image of voice into a convincing rendition of nationalist voice, so this full embodiment of Nazi life and national identity ultimately speaks its repressed subtext of corporal violence and sacrifice through decomposition. If the flayed female hand is a deathly image brought to life as fetish at the turn of the century, the overinvestment of signifiers of "life" is here transformed by history into an iconic representation of the deadly force that may aggregate in the medical gaze upon life.

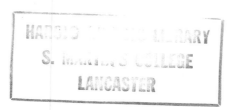

CHAPTER 6

Women and the Public Culture of Radiography

IN PREVIOUS CHAPTERS MY FOCUS was primarily on the subjectivity of the technician and the status of the body as object under the medical gaze. In this final chapter, I turn my attention directly to the communities and individuals who are imaged within that gaze. I consider the way that one social group, women, not only have been analyzed through X rays but have contributed in complex and conflicting ways to the establishment of a popular X-ray culture. I stated at the outset of this book that my concern here is the intertext between popular and professional techniques for organizing and transforming the body and cultural identity. The battery of new optical treatments under development in medicine are part of a visual culture that extends far beyond the field of medicine—a culture that includes the techniques of ultrasound, PET, MRI, and SPECT imaging. With these techniques in mind, I take up the following consideration of mass X-ray screening campaigns at midcentury.[1]

A recent controversy over federal funding of breast cancer research raises some important questions about gender and the national politics of high-tech imaging. In 1992, Congress earmarked $25 million in army money for 1993 breast cancer research. The Department of Defense (DOD) spent the entire sum on optical and locational detection devices: it outfitted the army, navy, and air force with stereotaxic mammography machines (computer-driven locational devices that zero in on the tiniest lump with great precision); it purchased new mammography equipment for U.S. bases in Pearl Harbor and Iceland; and it initiated a study of digital mammography and other experimental diagnostic methods. Meanwhile, responding to lobbying from the powerful National Breast Cancer Coalition (NBCC), Congress more than doubled previous allocations for breast cancer research, to $274 million. However, the increase exceeded a designated cap on domestic spending. Congress's solution was to direct only a small portion of the money ($64 million) to an agency with a demonstrated commitment to breast cancer research (the National Cancer Institute), rerouting the remaining $210 million into the defense budget. This move effectively placed the army in charge of what may be the most extensive federally funded breast cancer research program to date.[2]

The U.S. Army, an institution with a demonstrated lack of interest in women's rights, has been charged with researching a disease that kills about forty-six thousand U.S. women each year. Why this federal designation of the Department of Defense as guardian of women's health? This conflation of national defense and defense against disease is more than a little disturbing. Indeed, recent events suggest that, when the military has considered women at all, it has targeted them as objects of sexual conquest.[3] Perhaps it is not surprising, then, that, charged with the mission of researching a disease that affects the breast, that most erotically charged part of women's bodies, the army would choose to invest its $25 million in body imaging and locational devices, those techniques that emphasize visuality and the fetishization of the breast. Many breast cancer activists are arguing that this narrow focus on detection shortchanges research in such crucial areas as possible environmental and societal factors and genetic susceptibility. As breast cancer surgeon and NBCC activist Susan Love argues, "Mammography screening is certainly an important tool, but early detection is not prevention. The DOD agenda must move on."[4] Despite such objections, the DOD publicly stated that it is quite satisfied by its investment in imaging and locational technologies, and it will continue to invest in high-tech diagnostic equipment and research.

Accounts of the new medical imaging technologies in professional and popular media almost invariably invoke cases demonstrating the high payoff of imaging research. What is less frequently noted, however, is that in the United States the post–World War II ascendancy of imaging technologies in federally funded research and private medicine has been paralleled by a startling series of technological devolutions in imaging in the sphere of public health. The state of medical imaging in the late twentieth century might be described more accurately as two intersecting trajectories: private-sector medicine moving toward the routine use of high-end technologies, and public-sector health care in technological regression. The latter condition can be illustrated by some of the recent press surrounding the use of X rays in tuberculosis and breast cancer screening and diagnosis.

With the resurgence of epidemic TB since the late 1980s, many public clinics recently were set up or reopened in New York City boroughs to accommodate low-income people in need of diagnosis and treatment. At the nine clinics run by the New York City Health Department, many X-ray machines used for diagnosis and screening were reportedly broken or outdated (a 1991 *New York Times* article describes a "khaki green model with the levers and dials of an older era").[5] Where equipment was out of service, patients were sent to clinics in other boroughs, with crucial delays in detection; where it was outdated, image quality was unreliable and radiation was higher. While one might reason that resurrecting old equipment is acceptable in a crisis, such optimism is not warranted here—especially when newer technology is available in private medicine and research settings. This instance of active technological underdevelopment in U.S. public health has immediate consequences not only for the disenfranchised communities that TB has affected in disproportionate numbers, but for the (mostly female) technologists working in municipal health settings who are subject to high radiation levels as well as the frustrations of working with nonfunctioning or malfunctioning equipment.

The contradictions emerging in the scene of medical imaging are perhaps more clearly illustrated by a second crisis recently in the news, this one reported initially in a 1990 document from the New York City Office of the Comptroller and then publicized in *The Village Voice.* In its report "Poverty and Breast Cancer in New York City," the office reveals that the city's eleven municipal hospitals had no overall policy or comprehensive program on breast cancer detection for the low-income women who had to rely on the municipal system for health care. Only three of these hospitals offered mammography screening, and then only on a limited basis—to regular patients in their medical clinics, after long delays. Those using the facility were subject to inadequate image analysis and case follow-up. The city hospital system's patient death rate from breast cancer was three times above the national average of 24 percent, a statistic that the report attributes almost entirely to the unavailability of an early detection mechanism in the city's public hospitals and to the dire lack of institutional support (staffing, maintenance) for the three existing mammography facilities.[6] A 1992 report from the comptroller's office, tellingly titled "Radiation out of Control," shows that the X-ray units in place around the city were found overwhelmingly to lack adequate maintenance and inspection.[7]

In short, at the moment that high-tech imaging has become a specialization in itself around which entire medical departments and industries have formed, some of the most basic of medical imaging procedures—X-ray screening for tuberculosis and breast cancer—are conducted with alarmingly retrograde equipment and methods in the public health sphere. When I draw on examples that illustrate institutional control over technology and the down side of technohistory, I do not mean to imply that technology is not to be trusted, or that Western medicine constructs a narrative of technological evolution to mask its own genocidal or gynocidal agendas. Rather, my intention is to unpack the densely interwoven set of conditions and circumstances that constructs the scene of medical imaging. The culture of visual technology is critically informed by discourses outside the institutional world of medicine's imaging "experts." We cannot overlook the impact of popular visual cultures, patients, and medical and media activists on medicine's new visual culture.

What follows is an attempt to historicize the way bodies are regarded within the public discourse of radiography. As a public technology, the X ray has played a part in public health that is both risky and useful. The situation of medical imaging raises the critical question: is a medical counterculture possible at the high end of the technological scale? Through the following consideration of X-ray technology in the context of public health campaigns against tuberculosis and breast cancer, I hope to show that although the new medical imaging technologies are without question being used as a form of surveillance and control of bodies and communities, it would be a mistake to represent these technologies as simply tools of social domination. Without question, knowledge and authority are exerted through the surveillant techniques of disease management; however, certain bodies are systematically excluded from this gaze. One's identity is defined, in part, in terms of one's position within or on the margins of a social body composed through a visual apparatus that operates in terms of both what it will not image and what it will. Though medicine may control the bodies and communities it images, it also offers imaging as a class and cultural privilege.

This chapter will address two specific problematics. The first is the representation of women in the film media campaign against tuberculosis from the late 1930s to the middle 1950s. My main focus will be the promotion of the chest X ray, one of the key techniques used in the national campaign to monitor and control TB. The second is the slow and uneven technological experimentation in X-ray screening for breast cancer, and the incorporation of X-ray mammography in national public health institutions. These two problematics converge: despite the success, by the late 1940s, of the mass campaign to institute chest X ray for TB screening and diagnosis, X-ray screening for breast cancer was barely imagined until the early 1960s. Although women figure prominently in TB public health media, this presence is an inverse indicator of the wider regard for women's health during these years. Women appear in TB public health media not as the privileged objects of medical concern but as representative bearers of contagious and insidiously hidden infection. They play a metaphorical role as deceptive carriers of a disease that is invisible except under the X ray, threatening the integrity of the family, the community, and the nation. The technique of X ray, often presented in these films as a means of uncovering TB infection in the absence of visible signs and symptoms, is linked to a sexualized public surveillance of the body. Yet, while chest X ray was promoted as a means of publicly assessing the private interior of the body—a space persistently characterized in these films as feminine—X-ray imaging of the female breast as a cancer screening technique was barely a glimmer in the radiological researcher's imagination. During this period of intensive optical management of a vast sector of the population, the use of X ray in breast cancer diagnosis was subject to a puzzling lack of optical regard.[8]

Medicine's Public Gaze: Women in the TB Public Health Film

Women were disproportionately the protagonists and/or targeted viewers of the numerous motion pictures that were produced between the late 1930s and the middle 1950s to promote public knowledge about tuberculosis. This was not because women's health was a special concern of the medical and public health professions, nor because it was acknowledged that women were disproportionately affected by TB. Rather, women were regarded as domestic caregivers in charge of family and community health—as wives, mothers, housekeepers, and nurses. On one level, the media campaign against TB targeted the home as its main battleground and, by extension, women as key agents of disease control. Thus, although women had an unusual degree of agency in public health culture, their position was narrowly circumscribed. On another level, these films also identify the female body as a key vector of TB contagion. Carelessly infecting lovers, family, and community, the tubercular woman featured in many of the TB public health films of this period is an insidious threat to the public. She is dangerous not simply because she suffers from TB, but because she may spread the infectious disease without exhibiting its signs and symptoms.[9] The X ray, penetrating the opaque surface of the body to display previously imperceptible evidence of disease, is critically implicated in inscribing the private interior of the body within a surveillant gaze that makes disease both visible and public.

Tuberculosis, the most common cause of death in the United States and much of western Europe throughout the nineteenth century, initially was attributed to inherited constitutional weakness and unhealthy habits or environments. The identification of the tubercle bacillus microorganism in 1882 bolstered the view of TB as a contagious disease and not an inherent condition. By the twentieth century, it was broadly regarded as communicable and therefore confinable through extended monitoring and management of large populations. Public officials, philanthropists, and some physicians launched a national public health campaign to gauge, regulate, and control the activities of people with TB as a means of preventing or containing transmission. In the United States, the antituberculosis campaign's institutional apparatus included a battery of surveillance techniques: mandatory case reporting, statistical record keeping, educational media programs, and the formation of regulatory institutions (the TB sanitarium). There were no tested and effectively marketed treatment drugs for tuberculosis until midcentury. Nevertheless, as the physician Desmond Callan points out, TB incidence in the United States began to decline long before these antibiotics hit the market. Epidemiologists credit the decline to reductions in poverty and overcrowded housing—and to vigorous public health control measures.[10] Techniques of surveillance, involving the popularization of X-ray technology, thus remained the primary public health strategy until treatment drugs became available in the early 1960s.[11]

A 1991 entry in the *Morbidity and Mortality Weekly Report: Centers for Disease Control Surveillance Summaries* notes that the number of reported tuberculosis cases has been growing nationally since 1988, with a 9.4-percent increase in TB cases in 1989 (the largest annual increase to that date since 1953), and with disproportionately greater increases in reported cases occurring among their designated categories of Hispanics, non-Hispanic blacks, and Asians/Pacific Islanders, and among those in the age group twenty-five to forty-four.[12] (This increase is attributable in part to the rising number of tuberculosis cases among people with AIDS, whose compromised immune systems may leave them especially vulnerable to opportunistic diseases such as TB.) The relatively brief period of time between the supposed containment of TB nationally and what is being billed as its return indicates that the disease has continued to be endemic not only to Third-World countries or underdeveloped regions (for example, in sub-Saharan Africa, where TB is acknowledged as a persistent leading cause of death), but to Western metropolitan centers. Indeed, in some sectors of the United States (in poor urban communities or in migrant labor camps, for example), TB cases currently exceed those of the poorest countries in the world. As Peter Davis and John McKinlay argue, "a far more likely explanation for the resurgence of tuberculosis in the inner cities of the developed world is the reappearance of just these living conditions that the social and economic policies of the modern welfare state were designed to eliminate."[13]

Long believed to be most readily transmitted through the breathing of airborne particles which become trapped in high concentrations in unventilated spaces, or through contact with an infected person's sputum, tuberculosis has been associated historically with the often close and unventilated quarters of the urban poor and working class. Women, held responsible for domestic tasks such as sanitizing bedding and dishes and airing out rooms, were regarded as the family members chiefly responsible for the control of TB infection in the home. In a much-publicized lecture of 1903, the eminent physician William Osler identified the home as the critical site of TB infection and control:

> In its most important aspects the problem of tuberculosis is a home problem. In an immense proportion of cases the scene of the drama is the home; on its stage the acts are played, whether to the happy issue of recovery, or the dark ending of a tragedy, so commonplace as to have dulled our appreciation of its magnitude.[14]

Osler characterized the home not as a private sphere, but as a public theater for the staging of the familiar contagion narrative: the home is "the scene of the drama." Elsewhere, he characterized the home as a different kind of public theater—as a "battleground" for the war against disease. The medical historian Barbara Bates notes that "by calling for war in the home—the center of a woman's domain—Osler was sending a challenge to women."[15] Indeed, women could read this more accurately as an ultimatum: sanitize your home or risk your life. Even paid TB sanitarium and home care was designated women's work. It is therefore not surprising that in the many public health films produced and exhibited during the midcentury media campaign against TB, women were both the targeted viewers and the chief protagonists of a drama that was often set in the domestic "public theater."

Most of the public health films of the late 1930s through the middle 1950s feature white working-class women. However, the medical historian Edward H. Beardsley suggests that public health officials had statistics from 1940 showing that black women contracted TB at four to five times the rate of white women.[16] This situation was widely attributed not to economic and public health policies, but to African American communities' own "unhealthy" lifestyles.[17] The consequences of African American communities' purported failure to comply with modern public health measures is the subject of the 1938 narrative *Let My People Live*, a film in which a poor black southern woman—a character who never appears on screen, but is constantly invoked—is blamed for jeopardizing the health of her children and her community. She treats her TB symptoms at home with traditional remedies and ultimately dies, but not before infecting one of her children. Women's caretaking in the home is the source of transmission: Mary, the daughter who cares for her sick mother at home, is infected. George, who is away getting an education at the Tuskegee Institute, is spared. In an anguished postfuneral confession to her clergyman that assumes a link between tuberculosis transmission and biology, Mary admits that she herself is ill with what must surely be TB: "They say it runs in the family" (figure 6.1). The minister explains germ theory and directs Mary to a physician. But on her trip to the doctor's office, she is waylaid by a friend who says (quite accurately, and with a southern accent that is markedly distinct from Mary's northern diction), "Girl, ain't no doctor in the world that can cure you of tuberculosis." She recommends instead her own grandmother's herbal remedies. Mary discredits the knowledge of the girl's grandmother and her own mother as she dismisses her darker-skinned friend: "My mother believed in that—roots, herbs, and teas. I got to see Doctor Gordon." Mary, whose light skin symbolizes her assimilationist role in the narrative, survives because she submits to a diagnostic X ray and agrees to be placed in a TB sanitarium, a place where her disease, now made public, can be contained and monitored.

Through a narrative appeal bolstered by music from the Tuskegee Choir, *Let My People Live* represents community medicinal practice as a genocidal threat. This message is repeated in such films as *Another to Conquer*, the National Tuberculosis Association's 1941 dramatization of TB transmission in a Navajo community. Though never present on screen, Mary's mother and her friend's grandmother embody the insidious threat of disease and death posed by women's noncompliance with public health management and surveillance, as well as women's resistance to modern medicine in their use of traditional remedies and knowledges.

Whereas *Let My People Live* constructs a narrative of maternal culpability, the 1940 film *They Do Come Back* ties tuberculosis to a more sexually charged domestic contagion drama. A young white working-class man of "Everytown" suffers an oral hemorrhage. Tests reveal that he has TB, an illness whose source is proclaimed to be "lip contact" with his fiancée, who is identified as an asymptomatic carrier. The engulfing threat of "lip contact" is graphically dramatized in *You Can Lick TB*, a 1949 educational film produced by the Veterans Administration for men with the disease. In one shot, the hapless protagonist, Bill, hunches in the corner of the frame, dwarfed by an enormous pair of lipstick-covered lips that are superimposed on his image. Bill's doctor chides in voice-over: "TB germs. They didn't just happen. You got them from contact with somebody who already had TB." These monstrous lips, symbolizing the potent dangers of unauthorized sexual contact with women, threaten to kill every man (figure 6.2).

Mass TB screening entailed the institution of a public medical surveillance system that was both broad in scope and gauged to the minute and internal anatomical parts of the individual body. In the course of its narrative, *They Do Come Back* includes instructional sequences on what the young man should have done before risking the potentially deadly kiss (for one thing, the film suggests, he should have had his fiancée screened). As *Diagnostic Procedures in Tuberculosis*, a 1938 educational film for medical students, makes clear, mass screening techniques were advocated not because they prevented disease from occurring in the individual, but because they helped to institute public modes of surveillance and community prophylaxis across and among larger social groups (families, the workplace, communities). In this sense, the chest X ray, although reputed to identify TB in asymptomatic subjects, was by no means regarded as a preventive measure—not for the individual screened, at least. Rather, it functioned as a kind of *collective* prophylaxis, making identifiable the disease in its early stages and thus facilitating surveillance and separation of the tubercular subject from family or community.[18]

Let My People Live and *They Do Come Back* suggest that women were regarded not only as vectors of disease but also as privileged bearers of an infection characterized in its early stages by an insidious lack of visible signs. The potential for disease lay dangerously hidden and invisible within the nurturing and/or seductive female body. The woman's body symbolizes the threat of contagion, making quite literal the potential threat posed by the capacity of TB to be transmitted in the absence of any visible object or sign. The X ray is a particularly charged site of public surveillance and control, then, not only of women's bodies but of members of a public bearing a

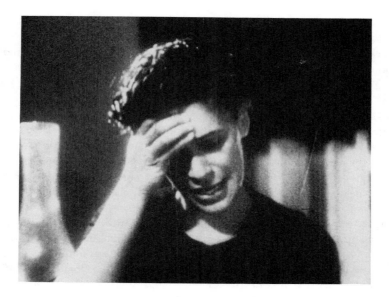

Figure 6.1. Mary confesses to her minister that she has tuberculosis. From *Let My People Live* (1938).

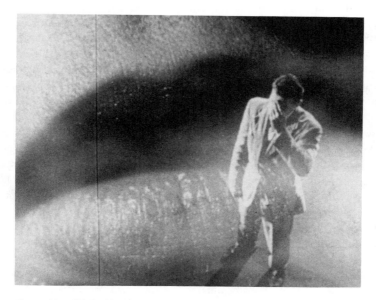

Figure 6.2. Bill licked by TB after some dangerous lip contact in *You Can Lick TB* (1949).

"feminine" capacity to transmit unseen infection. The chest X ray, bringing to sight the signs of disease that could not be seen on the surface of the body, thus becomes a critical medium precisely because it makes public each individual's private, internal state of health. Certainly this was not the first time that medicine had drawn the interior of the body into a visual signifying system.[19] But the institution of the TB chest X ray is of special significance for at least two reasons. First, it marks the entry of a visual technology of mass culture into the private domain of the individual body on a very large social scale. Like other emergent visual technologies of mass culture, such as television, the chest X ray had by midcentury become both a routine and a significant part of national life. The mass X-ray screening drew the private spheres of home and body into the purview of public culture. Second, the tuberculosis chest X ray implicated a mass visual technology in the project of community prophylaxis. Imaging is implicated not so much in representing the body as in preventing contagion across bodies, communities, and the nation.

The X-ray image constitutes a surveillant gaze that was not limited to the agency and authority of the medical doctor working in a laboratory or clinic. With the popularization of screening in a range of public health venues, the X ray was promoted and managed by radiological technologists, nurses, sanitarium superintendents, patients, and community members. Though some physicians strongly advocated X-ray screening for TB as early as 1910, it was not until 1926 that the X ray was widely regarded as "the pivotal point of early diagnosis and the guide and index of effective treatment in tuberculosis."[20] Surveillance in the form of the mobile screening unit and routine X-ray screening during hospital admissions procedures was instituted on a mass scale after 1936. But for these strategies to be effective, large numbers of people had to be convinced to trust, and even welcome, X-ray imaging. Promotional shorts produced by national tuberculosis organizations were often subsidized by corporations eager to generate a market for the technologies they manufactured. Through multiply sponsored films, routine TB screening of apparently healthy subjects was promoted on a mass scale as a safe, easy, and even pleasurable experience—just one among many positive, healthy experiences one might have with popular media culture in daily life.

Target TB, a 1950 public health film whose sponsors included General Electric, a manufacturer of X-ray equipment as well as home appliances, illustrates the media strategies used to engage women in the tuberculosis screening campaign. To demonstrate the havoc that TB wreaks in the body's interior, the film conflates perceived threats of national invasion and invasion of the individual body by disease. In a sequence of the film demonstrating modes of infection, we see an animated cartoon character, a Japanese soldier, infiltrating the body. The soldier infects the lungs by piercing their interior surface with his bayonet (figure 6.3). We are then shown a microscopic view of a tubercle which, in this film, coincidentally resembles the graphic design

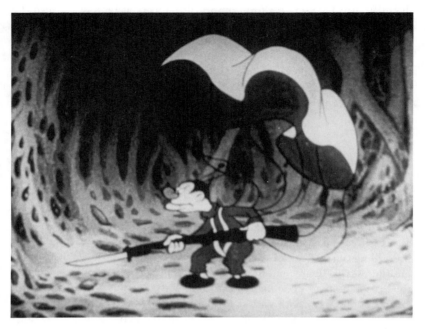

Figure 6.3. A "Japanese" soldier invading the body to infect it with TB. From *Target TB* (1950).

that adorns Japan's flag. Having established disease as an issue of national security, the film moves on to an instructive narrative about the agency of women in this matter of national security. We see a young white working-class woman and her coworkers venture with some trepidation into a mobile TB screening unit. The woman submits to her first-ever chest X ray, which is administered by a female nurse. Afterward, she remarks, "Why, that's as easy as having your picture taken." The nurse responds reassuringly, suggesting that X-ray imaging has it over snapshot portraiture: "It's simpler—you don't have to worry about getting the sun in your eyes." It is possible to argue that this scene represents women (including those with medical training) as naively unaware of the critical differences between X-ray technology and photographic optics. The X ray, a register of the passage of activated electrons through the field of the body, provides something quite different from the light imprint of the body surface. Far from a photograph of the body's interior appearance (the skeleton, the organs), the X ray is a record of variations in density throughout different regions of the body—a graphic image void of the familiar signifiers of difference attached to the surface appearance of the body encoded in the photograph. But there is another way to read this view of the X ray as snapshot portrait, a reading that undercuts the view that the X ray is a form of specialized technical looking. *Target TB* also suggests that X ray is an everyday form of imaging, a routine that women find easy and even pleasurable to participate in—both as imaged object and as imaging subject. The gaze in which these two women participate is authorized not only by their own consenting participation as imager and imaged but by a public culture that has made that gaze mobile and accessible, bringing it out of the medical institution and into the public space of the community.

Radiography's Mass Appeal: The Healthy Gaze

Although radiology was practiced almost exclusively by men in its first decades, women's bodies were often the test objects of early imaging research. I have argued (chapter 5) that the press's representation of the X ray as sexualized spectacle and as a new mode of illicit looking was not at all a misreading of the work of science but a foregrounding of the fact that visual pleasure, sexual desire, and the thrill of mortality were not just incidental to the male radiologist's conquest of the inner body.[21] It was precisely this association of the X ray both with sexual looking and with death that had to be managed in the promotion of this technique to the public in the midcentury TB screening campaign. The management involved a dual strategy: rendering public and surveillant the voyeuristic gaze of the male radiologist, and reencoding the private body as a public space that might be traversed by anyone—even women technologists. This dual agenda involved a transformation of the X ray from iconic death image to symbol of community health. *Target TB*'s alignment in 1950 of the X-ray image with *snapshot* photography, a mass-market technology through which consumers could produce images of themselves by themselves, marks the success of this campaign to supplant the experience of subjection to scientific voyeurism with participation in mass surveillance as a healthy mode of sexualized looking.

Highlights and Shadows, a 1937 Kodak Research Laboratories promotional film by James Sibley Watson Jr., a filmmaker-radiographer whose work was considered in the previous chapter, includes a sequence on X-ray technology that clearly illustrates this agenda. A mummy case removed from a tomb in Egypt is X-rayed in the Metropolitan Museum of Art laboratory, so that its entire contents are made, in the words of the film's narrator, "visible without the removal of a single wrapping." A shot of a laboratory technician operating X-ray equipment cuts to an X-ray image of the mummified skeleton. This is followed by a cut in to a medium shot of the mummy's head and chest in X ray, which dissolves into a matched shot of a drawing of an Egyptian head and torso (apparently the design imprinted on the mummy case exterior). This image is followed by a frontal shot of a young and attractive white woman, framed and positioned in medium close-up to duplicate exactly the pose of the drawn figure in the previous shot. A white man in a white lab coat steps into the frame and grasps the woman's head in his hands, forcing it sideways, effectively short-circuiting her gaze out toward the camera. The mummy sequence is then duplicated in reverse: a medium shot of the woman cuts to a full shot, in which we see that she is strapped tightly to a laboratory table and is wearing a swimsuit, into the bodice of which is tucked a large flower. Her photographic image gives way to a graphically matched body X ray, an image that the camera scans, taking in the whole body X ray in a quick vertical tilt. Nothing so much as an assessing once-over glance is evoked as the camera takes in all of this "sexy" skeleton. Over this last shot, as the musical score that accompanies this sequence rises in crescendo, the film's male narrator announces that "this young lady, to whom henceforth a glass house should hold no terrors, will, after an examination of her radiographs, be reassured that she is *indeed* physically fit" (figure 6.4).

The narrator of *Highlights and Shadows* asserts the transformation of "this young lady's" potential fears not only of exposure to radiation, but of exposure to the radiographer's penetrating look into the body. It is significant that this sequence's apparent project of desensitizing viewers to the radiologist's gaze rhetorically links the "private" interior space of the female body to the exposed domestic space of the "glass house." This "house" is here the female body's exterior, a protective epidermis that yields under the optical pressure of the X ray. The sequence suggests that the "terror" of exposing one's private spaces to public judgment metaphorically implied in the adage is linked to (feminine) "terror" of exposing one's private interior to the radiographer's assessing glance. Like the occupant of the glass house, the subject of the X ray is vulnerable because regions of her body usually kept private are placed on display. But this vulnerability to sight is transformed into a condition of health. The idea of making public her bodily interior should "hold no terror" for the "young lady" whose swimsuit-clad body is already exposed, and whose chest X ray further confirms "that she is *indeed* physically fit." Here health is aligned with particular cultural conventions of femininity and beauty: the woman who is "fit" is white, young, and conventionally pretty—and she enjoys having her picture taken. The conflation of woman and mummy underscores the point that the X ray, far from a technology of death and bodily decomposition, in fact preserves (or mummifies) the woman in her youthful "fitness." But it also evokes the specter of the vampiric tubercular woman and the insidious threat of contagion (through "lip contact," for example) that may lie beneath the seductively fit exterior of any woman.

This sequence from *Highlights and Shadows* hints at transformations of meaning incumbent on the introduction of the X ray into the sphere of public health. First, the X ray, regarded as an icon of death in the popular press

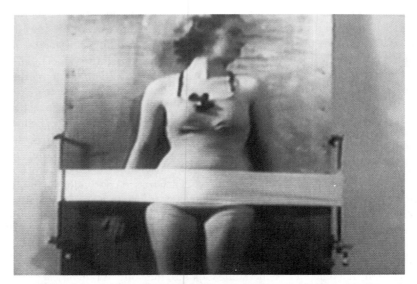

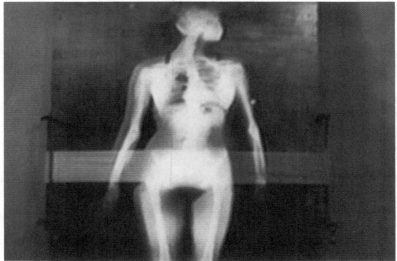

Figure 6.4. Frames from *Highlights and Shadows* (1937).

at the turn of the century and later, has been transformed by midcentury into an icon of health and life. Second, sexualized and racialized standards of beauty and health, conventionally inscribed onto the surface of the body (the appearance of skin color and visage, for example), are now encoded in interior qualities—in the state of the lungs, the skeletal system, and so on. The X

ray vies with the photograph as a new cultural register of identity and difference. But for the X ray to be embraced widely as an indexical register of
identity and difference, it had to be embraced as a source of potential identification among its public. As Anne Friedberg has noted with respect to cinematic images, identification requires a recognizable or normative body
figure/image.[22] The reversing of the X ray's iconic status as unauthorized
death-image was critical in the encoding of the X-ray image as a normative
model of the healthy body.

The campaign to effect this public transformation of the X ray among the
working class is nowhere more evident than in *Mass Radiography*, a 1944
British government instructional film that teaches industrial managers and
workers about the benefits of instituting industrial workplace X-ray screening. This film is one of a number of similar films produced in the United
States and England to model mass X-ray screening in plants and factories. It
takes the viewer through the steps of equipment setup, mass worker screening, image analysis, and follow-up of suspected TB cases. This film's narrative centers on Mary, a young, white, and blonde factory worker who, like
the woman in *Target TB*, has reservations about getting X-rayed. Mary is introduced at work, narcissistically gazing at her own image mirrored in the
polished metal surface of the machinery she operates, as she listens to a female voice on the loudspeaker dictate the procedure for the mandatory
screening process. As we are taken through the steps of the screening, we see
female technologists conducting X rays of men and women alike. By the end
of the film, we see that Mary has come to accept the full benefits of X-ray
culture: she presents her lover with two framed portraits, a photograph of
her face and an X-ray image of her chest, both signed "To Tom with all my
love, from Mary" (figure 6.5). As the camera pans from one image to the
other, the male voice-over confirms the implied address to female workers,
as well as their supposed desire to be looked at and to be authorized as safe
objects of male desire: "For you," he says, an X ray "means that someone can
say not only 'Sure she's pretty,' but 'Sure she's healthy.'"

An important component of the mass X-ray campaign, popular science
newsreel sequences also invited women to enjoy being the object of a new
mode of visual culture, to recognize the X-ray image as a gauge of gender
and sexual identity, and even to identify with it narcissistically. *The Inside
Story*, a newsreel about visual technologies across a spectrum of disciplines,
produced in the 1950s for prefeature movie-house entertainment, uses X-
ray motion studies to expose hidden signs of sexual attraction in an apparently platonic encounter. A couple is pictured in moving X ray sipping from
teacups, the fluid they ingest visibly sliding down their throats. The male
narrator states in jovial voice-over that "tea with a dash of barium" (a radiographic contrast medium) is being served to "Miss Jones" and "Mr. Smith"
at the Hotel Deluxe, where they are enjoying the performance of a classical

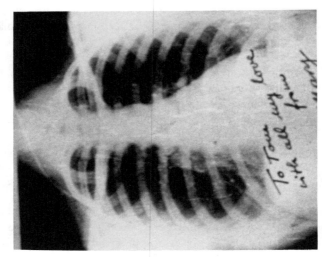

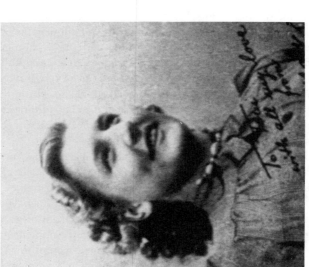

Figure 6.5. Mary's snapshot portraits, from *Mass Radiography* (1944).

music ensemble, whose performance we witness in X ray and sync sound.[23] We are also given a sync-sound view of Mr. Smith's heart, which, the narrator informs us, is beating "at a normal clip." We then see this same heart beating frantically—a change that occurs, we are told, in response to the image we have only just seen of Miss Jones's lungs (a not insignificant choice of organs) as she sighs in pleasure over the musical performance of the skeletal ensemble. "Mr. Jones tries to be nonchalant," the narrator explains, "but his heart beating twice as fast as it should be marks him as a dead duck." The sequence sets up a surveillant gaze in which the narrator—clearly coded as comedian, not scientist—invites the audience to participate in the public exposure of hidden signs of sexual desire to a mass cinema audience. Gender difference marks this surveillant gaze: as the case of Mr. "Dead Duck" Smith shows, the erotic spectacle of Miss Jones's lungs is enough to kill a man. In this sequence, the interior of the body—and notably the lungs, the critical site of TB's definitive visibility—becomes erotically charged, as a site of sexual and pathological knowledge. A previously generic set of organs like the lungs is invested with the power to incite visual pleasure precisely because it has become a privileged site of knowledge about illness and death.

Clearly, the stripping away of flesh in these films in no way implies a dissolution of the cultural markers of sexual difference. A Paramount newsreel of the same period underscores this message. In this film, a conventional moving image of a woman applying lipstick dissolves into X ray. But stripping away the gender-encoded face and hair fails to strip the signs of gender from the scene: the X-ray image renders all the more clearly the woman's jewelry, metal lipstick tube, and compact, all items made of X-ray-resistant materials. Like the popular turn-of-the-century X-ray photograph of the female hand with only the bones and metal wedding ring visible, and like the Rochester film of a woman "applying" the means of her own visibility by applying face makeup, the cinematic X-ray image becomes a means of reinforcing the cultural signs of gender and sexual difference.

The Visual Culture of Mammography

Researchers in breast cancer diagnosis and screening often characterized the breast as an elusive object that actively eluded attempts at standardized screenings through qualities encoded as "feminine." The breast was characterized as too soft, too irregular in composition, and too changeable to image clearly. Radiography makes images of variations in density through sections of the body composed of bone or relatively hard tissue. It is not suited to imaging of the breast, a region composed of fluid, soft tissue. Rather than adapt the technology to its object (or to the dominant perception of its object), radiologists more often attempted to adapt the breast to the technique.

In the relatively few cases of breast imaging research conducted before 1960, radiographers sliced, compressed, or halted physiological change in the breast in an attempt to bring it in line with the X ray. In short, women's bodies were regarded as inherently resistant to a technology that could save women's lives.

It is estimated that a U.S. woman's odds of getting breast cancer now stand at one in eight, double the odds of 1940; however, the recent surge in cases may be due precisely to better detection mechanisms such as mammography, rather than to a higher incidence rate.[24] Breast cancer screening and diagnosis have been at the center of discussions about these data. Like TB treatment and screening, X-ray mammography has been an object of close scrutiny in recent years because it is the only method widely tested and made available to large numbers of women for breast cancer screening and diagnosis—that is, aside from the invaluable low-tech method of breast self-examination.

It was not until almost twenty years after the inception of radiography's use in medicine that the first report of a relatively extensive study of radiography of the breast was published.[25] This 1913 study centered on the X-ray analysis of breast tissue already surgically removed from women's bodies: the physician used X rays to analyze about three thousand mastectomy sections. Removed from the breast and cut into very thin slices, each tumor was evaluated with X-ray microscopy. This study, though confined to tiny flat slices of dead tissue, had some important implications for the identification and diagnosis of breast cancer in living bodies. It suggested that X-ray was a potentially accurate gauge of a tumor's composition. It is not a huge leap from this finding to the more far-reaching idea that the X ray might be used to confirm and accurately locate tumors in living bodies.

These findings, though clearly indicating the potential for X-ray screening and diagnosis, were not pursued for more than a decade. The author of a recent volume on the history of radiography provides two explanations for this historical lack of interest: technical difficulty (the then-current technology produced images of poor quality) and the general acceptance of surgery as a diagnostic procedure.[26] The significance of the latter explanation cannot be underestimated. One team of breast radiography researchers writing in 1960 paraphrased the continued objections to X-ray diagnosis among their contemporaries: "'Why should we burden ourselves with the problems of roentgenological [radiographic] examination of the female breast? A biopsy is usually necessary and will give the diagnosis anyway.'"[27] Surprisingly, the noninvasive technique of breast radiography was viewed as a redundant measure well into the 1950s and early 1960s, a period when research for the sake of knowledge was a booming business—moreover, a period when imaging was becoming a critical part of the medical knowledge-production business.

This reluctance regarding breast X ray underscores medicine's historical lack of regard for diseases that occur primarily in women. This point was made implicitly by an advocate of breast radiography research in the late 1950s. This physician admonished his colleagues for not treating the signs of breast cancer with the seriousness that they would the signs of, not surprisingly, tuberculosis:

> There is no thought of omitting roentgen [X-ray] study of the chest in an individual with hemoptysis [the coughing up of blood] and a positive sputum [test for TB]. There similarly should be no hesitation to obtain whatever additional information may be made available by a roentgen breast examination despite the clarity of the clinical picture. Completely unsuspected pathology may be uncovered.[28]

This directive that there should be no shortcuts taken in the diagnosis of breast cancer implies that such shortcuts were indeed being taken, and indicates that physicians rationalized the lack of attention to illnesses more common among women even in cases where diagnosis involved a proven technology. Although as early as 1930 there was some indication that X-ray technology could be used for breast cancer diagnosis, there was no rush to dedicate radiological research to the study of the female breast. But this physician introduced an idea that was not yet widespread: that X ray might identify *unsuspected* cancers—in other words, that it might be used to screen for cancer in apparently healthy subjects. It is this possibility that was elided by surgeons seeking to bypass breast radiography and go straight to surgery.

It was by chance that X ray had been researched for breast cancer diagnosis nationally in the 1930s. While trying to standardize techniques for X-ray analysis of the thoracic aorta, Stafford Warren, the radiologist who inaugurated X-ray cinema research at Rochester and the chief physician of the Manhattan Project, happened to note that the breast was silhouetted on the image. Seeing the potential diagnostic value of his images, he did some research.[29] Warren's study is significant in that it focused specifically on breast cancer diagnosis in living women's bodies rather than on classification of already excised tumors. Initially, there was great interest in his technique when he reported an accuracy rate of 93 percent in the diagnosis of small tumors in 58 of the 119 patients he studied. Yet his project was not followed by any significant research until the late 1950s. In the paragraphs that follow, I consider some of the "obstacles" that the breast reputedly presented to future research.

In order to understand the perceived impediments to Warren's research, it is necessary briefly to recall the TB chest X ray. In the 1938 *Highlights and Shadows*, the woman is X-rayed not to diagnose a suspected illness, but to screen for signs of health (that is, the radiologist wants a picture of her fit lungs). The routine mass radiography scheme tacitly promoted to apparently healthy subjects in this brief sequence functioned to encourage people to obtain a baseline image of the lungs in their healthy state. But for Warren and his fellow researchers, even the healthy breast was not normal. They complained that the breast, constantly undergoing changes in density, structure, and shape not only over the course of a woman's life but over the course of the menstrual cycle, defied the very idea of a normal state.[30] In an attempt to get around this perceived problem, Warren used serial images (sometimes shot in motion picture film) to encode changes tied explicitly to what he designated women's "normal" physiological states (the menstrual cycle and pregnancy, for example). This emphasis on physiological change in the breast was not always tied to diagnosis but extended to the designation of change as a pathological condition in itself, critically linked to women's social and psychical states. This effect is apparent in another radiological team's typology of "the normal breast"—a 1930 study in which X-ray views illustrate the breast during developmental stages that include "the adolescent virginal breast" and "the postclimacteric and senile breast."[31] Indeed, instability continues to be identified in some medical literature as a condition predisposing "feminine" tissue (in the breast, the cervix, or the uterus, for example) to the pathological extremes of cellular change that mark the designated continuum of cancer.

I noted earlier that X-ray technology privileges flat or narrow regions of the body. A constant complaint of radiologists was that the technique's narrow field of focus prohibited adequate imaging of organs or zones characterized by significant density or volume, such as the female breast. Warren developed a stereoscopic technique to render the breast in 3-D X rays. However, his technique did not provide enough resolution and detail to discern tumors accurately. The current method of compressing the breast between Plexiglas plates in order to obtain sharper X-ray resolution demands consideration in terms of cultural anxieties around breast size and volume. At the very least, it raises the important question of why a technology developed precisely for imaging bone and hard tissue with little depth resolution is currently the standard technique—indeed, the only approved technique—for imaging a dimensional soft tissue mass. In the section that follows, I consider the place of the breast in the development of ultrasound, the locational technique adapted precisely for the imaging of soft tissue.

Ultrasound: The Breast as Test Object

It is by now commonly held that medical ultrasound had its origins in military systems used in World War II to locate submarines and other objects hidden below the surface of the ocean. As Rosalind Petchesky has noted in her important study of ultrasound in obstetrics, "most technologies in a militarized society either begin or end in the military," and ultrasound is no exception.[32] I want to stress here, however, that ultrasound technology was already in medical use well before the war—in the 1920s and 1930s as a therapeutic treatment (in the destruction of body-surface tumors, for example),[33] and in the 1930s as an internal-body imaging system. Before and during the war, two Viennese researchers, a physicist and a neurologist, devised a system whereby ultrasound waves were passed through the skull in a scanning pattern to register in an attenuated image on a photographic plate (much as a television image forms in a scanning process). By the late 1940s, the acoustics laboratory at the Massachusetts Institute of Technology conducted medical ultrasound research with funding from the navy. The study was not very successful because the brain, surrounded by hard bone, defied interrogation by reflecting a "noisy" array of indecipherable signals.[34] The breast, however, would prove to be a much more user-friendly test object.

Just after the war, John J. Wild of the University of Minnesota Department of Surgery, with the help of Donald Neal, a navy aerospace engineer, reoutfitted for medical use an ultrasound generator that had been a radar training device. Wild, whose technique was the basis for the linear and graphic "A-mode" of ultrasound currently used in only a very few applications (fetal cephalometry—the measurement of the fetal skull in utero—is one), conducted his earliest experiments not only on postmortem material (malignant brain tumors), but on living beings. Two of these living entities were healthy, "normal" objects: test animals and Wild's own arm. The third, the female breast, was chosen because it was regarded as inherently pathological and because it was conveniently composed and situated. A study of breast tumors in living women constituted the first ultrasound imaging research Wild conducted on a human body other than his own.

Wild's selection for his test object of breast tumors in living subjects is important not only because it seems to suggest that he may have recognized the dire need for a breast cancer diagnostic technique (recall that this was the early 1950s and X-ray mammography was not yet being considered seriously) but also because it indicates that he considered women's bodies an appropriate choice for his first full-scale test on humans. While Wild limited exposure of his body to an extremity, sparing the vital organs housed in the torso from any contact with ultrasonic vibrations, his research on women involved a region of the body close to vital organs like the heart and the lungs. At the time that Wild worked, very few researchers were risking exposure of human bodies to ultrasound; no one could be certain about the biological effects of exposure. Published in the same month as Wild's first report of his breast studies is an essay in which Wild, Neal, and a coauthor summarize ultrasound exposure tests conducted by a range of researchers.[35] All experiments but one focus on animal tests. The exception is a 1939 experiment, "Curious Effects of Ultrasound," a test conducted on a living woman. According to the summary by Wild and his colleagues of this very early experiment, the researcher "reported diminished mental capabilities occurring in a woman who was exposed to a 16,000 cycle ultrasonic source for an hour." Without noting the nature or extent of the woman's "diminished mental capabilities," the authors state that "the effects were reversible by removing her from the ultrasonic chamber."[36]

Why was a test on a human body (other than that of a researcher directly involved in the project) conducted as early as 1939; why was a woman chosen; and why was such extensive exposure administered? Without addressing these questions, Wild and his associates assure their readers that their own method of using pulsed rather than continuous vibrations produced no known biological effects. Curiously, they make no note of their own work with women's bodies during this period. A second March 1951 publication, by Wild and Neal, indicates the sequence of their work on humans.[37] This essay, which focuses on the use of ultrasound to detect changes of texture in living tissue, includes a section, "Possibility of Harmful Effects," in which the authors' first work on living human bodies is described. After explaining that the risks are not known, Wild and Neal state that "the arm of one of us was first used" to find out what they might be. A small, hand-held ultrasound transducer was applied to Wild's forearm for thirty minutes. He reports that he experienced no sensation of heat or pain, and the arm exhibited no signs of damage during the following eight months. Wild and his colleagues then proceeded directly to work on the breast.

No images were recorded in the arm experiment. As the authors explain, this was essentially a test of the effects of ultrasound on tissue, and not the reverse—that is, it was not a test to determine the effectiveness of tissue in reflecting "readable" wave patterns. However, the experiments on women's bodies that followed were conducted precisely to test the viability of ultrasound imaging. Wild and his coauthors apparently were well aware that the breast studies were dismissive of risk evaluation. In 1952 they preface a lengthy account of the breast studies with a summary of past work in risk evaluation (including the arm experiment), concluding this section with the following disclaimer:

> A cautious but positive approach to an area of the patient provided with sensory organs responsive to heat and pain, after all advantage has been taken of the experimental animal, is recommended for testing untried ultrasonic apparatus. *In the final test of safety, someone has to be the last link in the chain.* We consider our echographic studies to be concerned with the effects of tissue on sound, rather than the reverse.[38]

It is interesting that the authors would suggest that "someone" has to be the "last link" when Wild himself thus far had been both the last and the only human link in their chain of safety testing. Wild and his coworkers conducted tests not of safety but of "effects of tissue on sound" on his first human subjects, twenty-one women with breast tumors. The choice of women with possible cancers is misleading, because it suggests—wrongly— that the authors were motivated by an interest in the diagnostic potential of the technique. They make it quite clear, rather, that they are interested only in the assessment of their equipment. They state more than once that they are concerned strictly with "the effects of tissue on sound." This rendering gender neutral of the test object, "tissue," is meant quite literally. Explaining that they do not intend their work to replace "existing methods of diagnosis of breast lesions" (recall that the existing method in 1951 is biopsy!), they aver that the breast is a mere placeholder, studied "with a view to applications to other sites."[39]

This reluctance is striking because the authors' findings seem to indicate the real potential of ultrasound as a modality for breast-cancer screening. Wild's first experiments were conducted on two women (sixty-six and forty years old, respectively), both of them with palpable breast lumps. In the first case, the hand-held transducer was applied to a normal area of the breast, and two sonograms were recorded. The transducer then was shifted to the area over the nodule, and an image taken (figure 6.6). The report notes that an increased number and amplitude of echoes in the latter image could easily be discerned in a lump that, on biopsy, proved to be an adenocarcinoma 2.5 centimeters in size (a fairly advanced tumor).[40] The finding would seem to indicate great potential for ultrasound in breast cancer screening and diagnosis. But in the published records of this and subsequent studies by Wild and colleagues, no notice is taken of these implications. The authors' major report concludes with a recommendation for further inquiry, but given the stated focus of this inquiry on tissue's effects on sound it would be difficult to construe this advice as a call for more research on breast tumors. Composed of soft tissue unlikely to engender overly complex images and conveniently packaged in the body as a set—the adjacent breast providing a duplicate object that functioned quite conveniently as an experimental control or norm[41]—the breast served its purpose and then virtually disappeared from the ultrasonic scene for more than a decade.[42]

Like the development of X-ray mammography, that of ultrasound mammography is marked by long lapses in interest, research, and funding. It was not until the early 1980s that physicians and researchers gave the technology serious consideration.[43] Perhaps the greatest irony is that although ultrasound was first researched for fetal imaging after Wild's breast studies (in the late 1950s), by the eighties fetal imaging had become for many the definitive use of the technique while ultrasound mammography remained an experimental technique, even now considered useful only in exceptional cases (where a woman's breasts are too dense to image with clarity on an X ray, as is often the case for women under thirty-five, or to determine whether a mass is solid, and thus possibly cancerous; or fluid, and thus possibly a cyst). Signifi-

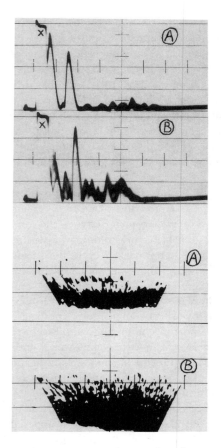

Figure 6.6. One–dimensional and two–dimensional ultrasound scans of the breast. In both sets, (A) represents a healthy breast and (B) a cancerous breast. From J. J. Wild, "Echographic Studies of Tumors of the Breast," *American Journal of Pathology* 28 (1952): 861.

cantly, Susan Love devotes less than a page of her breast-care manual to ultrasound mammography. While this near omission would seem to suggest that ultrasound breast screening has been proven ineffective, it is attributable to the fact that breast ultrasound research simply has not been adequately funded and pursued. Elizabeth Kelly-Fry, one of the few researchers in ultrasound mammography during the 1960s, concludes that

> the nature of some of the needed experiments [in ultrasound breast imaging] was such that they should have been carried out by physical science experts in the field of acoustics as a natural follow-up to the pioneer investigations [of Wild]. That such experiments were not pursued at an early date is partially related to the fact that the object in question is the female breast.[44]

Ultrasound was not the only technique that could potentially compete with the X ray for the market of breast tumor detection; several other experimental breast imaging techniques were considered roughly at the same time as

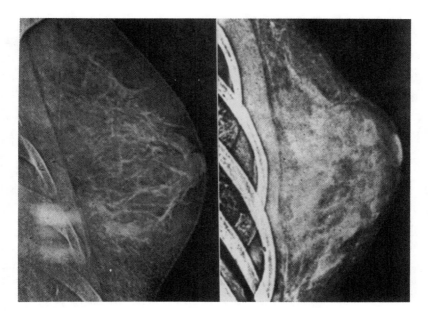

Figure 6.7. First xeromammography. From H. R. Gould et al., "Xerography of the Breast," *American Journal of Radiography* 84, no. 2 (1960): 222.

ultrasound. These include xeromammography, an institutionally accredited method developed by Xerox Corporation, which uses relatively high radiation (figure 6.7); thermography, a form of imaging that records temperature differences in areas of the body; transillumination, in which an intense light is passed through breast tissue to make a shadow image; and stereotaxic locational devices, which use computer-analyzed digital mammograms to locate the exact coordinates of a tumor and mechanically guide a biopsy needle in tumor aspiration procedures. More recently, magnetic resonance imaging is being considered as a screening technique.[45] But the majority of medical texts express pessimism and caution about these techniques (with the exception of xeromammography and stereotaxic methods), asserting that X ray is the reliable method. Kelly-Fry suggests that professional competition has been a major factor behind these misgivings. She explains that X-ray mammography underwent its first period of intensive research during precisely the period in which breast ultrasound was first actively researched (the 1960s); competition with X-ray mammography seemed to many a financially risky prospect. It is important to note here that in the 1960s research on X ray was limited to a comprehensive study by the Health Insurance Plan (HIP) of Greater New York. This was not a highly funded research project or a public health venture, but a health care corporation's investigation of a

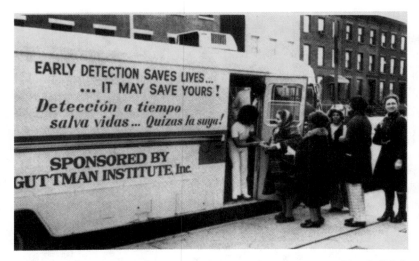

Figure 6.8. Mobile mammography unit used in the late 1960s. From R. H. Gold et al., "High-lights from the History of Mammography," *RadioGraphics* 10 (1990). Reprinted with permission of the Radiological Society of North America.

financially viable means of making screening available to a large number of middle- and working-class women. Like the advocates of mass X-ray screening for tuberculosis, HIP was motivated to come up with a mass screening system that would be both cost-effective and commercially viable for a vast number of users.[46] These attributes continue to be important in the development of new mammography technology. For example, the lag in research on ultrasound mammography is due in no small part to the economics of the technology industry (will ultrasound mammography undercut the X-ray market?) and to the economics of medical practices (what physician or clinic wants to carry the cost of reoutfitting the office with a whole new technology?). Consequently, although these days the private breast clinic usually has a dedicated ultrasound unit, the group health plan is lucky to have a lunking old dedicated X-ray unit. Hence, in the age of "new" imaging technologies, a hundred-year-old technique developed for imaging bone is the only breast screening option for most women (figure 6.8).

Conclusion

The HIP study of 1963 was a major turning point in X-ray mammography because it began to move mammography from private, experimental, and almost random use into the public sphere. It initiated the standardization of X-ray techniques, equipment, and modes of analysis (a critical step in making the technique available to a larger population); it marked the broad pop-ularization of the technique; and it set in motion the incorporation of mam-mography into the public health system, in theory making it accessible to low-income women. In critiquing the mechanisms, texts, and processes of the history of TB and breast cancer screening, I have tried to suggest that the trajectories of high and low technology are directed not only by professional interests but by public use, desire, and demand. In the public gaze that man-ages bodies and communities, women are implicated in roles beyond that of patient/victim. Following the example of ACT-UP (AIDS Coalition to Un-leash Power) and other politically effective AIDS activist and advocacy groups, many breast cancer activists—a group that includes women technol-ogists and physicians—are currently challenging professionally mandated modes of detection and research. Not only are they promoting that most ef-fective and underconsidered low-tech detection procedure, the breast self-exam, but they are promoting more intensive research in cause and prevention and broader distribution of high-tech detection devices. In order to carry out this work more effectively, I would argue, it is critical that we make strategic use of the models and warnings provided in the long and complex history of medical imaging technologies in public culture.

I return here to my claim that the public culture of prophylactic imaging that emerged around the mass X-ray screening campaign against tuberculosis constituted the emergence of a double-edged public gaze. I characterize this gaze as surveillant, but I do not suggest that surveillance is by necessity a to-talizing mode of institutional domination and control of populations. I de-scribe this gaze as a mode of perception whose agents are not only or primarily physicians and scientists but are also imaging technologists (the ma-jority of whom these days are women),[47] patients, and medical activists. I contrast this multivalent gaze to a male voyeuristic one that I argue is in place only partially, in the early decades of medical radiography and in some as-pects of the research process. I make this distinction because I want to show that contemporary medical imaging technologies, when viewed in their his-torical context, cannot simply be demonized as the optical tools of medical surveillance. At this point in history, there is too much at stake to condemn imaging technologies as militarized tools of social control. Without question, the gaze that constitutes the contemporary control and management of TB and breast cancer in the United States is organized in large part through a medical and public health bureaucracy. This gaze privileges populations that can afford private medical care, often subjecting those that cannot to humil-iating or damaging treatment or to no treatment at all.

It is important to note that few involved in the struggles against tubercu-losis and breast cancer are calling for eradication of medical technologies. Rather, the struggle is for equitable, affordable, and Medicare-covered access to existing technology; for high-end units in public as well as private medical settings; for increased supervision, maintenance, and trained staffing of equipment in public care settings; and for research on technologies' new uses for illnesses, like breast cancer, TB, and AIDS, that currently are afflicting primarily low-income women and other disenfranchised peoples.[48] Without question, knowledge, authority, and domination are exerted through a visual ordering of bodies; however, certain bodies (and certain body parts) are differently configured within, if not just excluded from, that gaze. As was suggested above, communities are thus defined, in part, in terms of their relative positions within or on the margins of a social body composed through a surveillant apparatus that operates as much through what it refuses to image as through what it fixes clearly in its sight. The point, then, is not that images constitute privileged medical knowledge and power over those imaged and therefore women should resist being imaged; rather, women must actively reconfigure technologies of representation—precisely because these technologies have been invested with the power to transform the body physically. Although medical imaging technologies may not be a cure, they are a critical—and heavily funded—area of visual culture. Thus this field is in need of active feminist technological refunctioning and countersurveillance.[49]

Notes

Introduction

1. Barbara Duden, *Disembodying Women: Perspectives on Pregnancy and the Unborn* (Cambridge: Harvard University Press, 1993), 1.

2. Foucault, *The Order of Things: An Archaeology of the Human Sciences* (New York: Vintage Books, 1973), 129–30. I consider this passage from Foucault at greater length in chapter 1.

3. This point is considered at greater length in subsequent chapters.

4. Terry Ramsaye, *A Million and One Nights: A History of the Motion Picture through 1925* (New York: Simon and Schuster, 1926), xxxvii–xxxviii.

5. Michel Foucault, *The Birth of the Clinic: An Archaeology of Medical Perception* (New York: Random House, 1975), 141.

6. Adolf Nichtenhauser, M.D., "A History of Motion Pictures in Medicine" (Bethesda, Md.: National Library of Medicine, History of Medicine Division, circa 1950).

7. Anthony Michaelis, *Research Films in Biology, Anthropology, Psychology and Medicine* (New York: Academic Press, 1955).

8. Fatimah Tobing Rony, "On Ethnographic Cinema: 'Race,' Science, and Spectacle, 1895–1933" (Ph.D. diss., Yale University, 1993).

1. Science and the Cinema

1. "Auguste Lumière: Death of a Great Scientist" (New York Academy of Medicine Biographical Pamphlet File: n.d.)

2. Edgar Morin's *Le cinéma; ou, L'homme imaginaire* begins with an analysis of the historical coincidence of the airplane and the Cinématographe. The term "Cinématographe" is used both to refer to the specific invention of the Lumière brothers and as a generic term for the many camera/projectors that appeared roughly simultaneously in the west in 1895 (the U.S. Vitascope, the British Animatograph, and the German Bioscope). The scientist Léon Bouly had already used the term in an 1892 French patent for a motion camera. See Robert Soulard on the "Cinématographe Bouly," *Revue d'Histoire des Sciences* 16 (1963): 317–22.

3. Auguste Lumière, *La recherche scientifique* (Paris: Société d'Edition d'Enseignement Superieur, 1948), 5.

4. Ibid., 5.

5. The lab also produced Lumière Allarol, a "scientific" toothpaste produced for the mass market and guaranteed to kill invisible microscopic flora. Many of Lumière's essays on experimental physiology appear in the in-house publication in which the ads for this toothpaste appear, the *Annales des Laboratoires à Lumière de physiologie expérimentale et de pharmacodynamie*, published between 1921 and 1939.

6. See C. W. Ceram, *Archaeology of the Cinema* (New York: Harcourt, Brace and World, 1965); Jacques Deslandes, *Histoire comparée du cinéma,* vol. 1, *De la cinématique au cinématographe* (Tournai, Belgium: Casterman, 1966); and Georges Sadoul, *Histoire générale du cinéma,* vol. 1 (Paris: Denoel, 1973).

7. On the science film genre, see F. A. Talbot, *Moving Pictures: How They Are Made and Worked* (London, 1912; New York: Arno Press, 1970). The cinema in medical research is the subject of an unpublished manuscript by Adolf Nichtenhauser, M.D., "A History of Motion Pictures in Medicine" (Bethesda, Md.: National Library of Medicine, History of Medicine Division, circa 1950), and Anthony Michaelis, *Research Films in Biology, Anthropology, Psychology, and Medicine* (New York: Academic Press, 1955).

8. Alan Williams, "The Lumière Organization and Documentary Realism," in *Film before Griffith,* ed. John Fell (Berkeley and Los Angeles: University of California Press, 1983), 158; emphasis in original.

9. Ibid.

10. Talbot, *Moving Pictures,* 18.

11. On the history of institutional photography as a mode of social regulation in the public sphere, see John Tagg, *Burdens of Representation: Essays on Photographies and Histories* (Minneapolis: University of Minnesota Press, 1993).

12. Some examples of technological-determinist histories of the early cinema are Michael Chanan, *The Dream That Kicks: The Prehistory and Early Years of the Cinema* (London and Boston: Routledge and Kegan Paul, 1980); Sadoul, *Histoire du cinéma mondiale: Des origines à nos jours* (1949; Paris: Flammarion, 1972); Raymond Fielding, *Technological History of Motion Pictures and Television* (1967; Berkeley and Los Angeles: University of California Press, 1983); and Gordon Hendricks, *Origins of the American Film* (New York: Arno Press, 1972).

13. Stephen Heath, "Technology as Historical and Cultural Form," in *The Cinematic Apparatus,* ed. Teresa de Lauretis and Stephen Heath (New York: St. Martin's Press, 1980), 1.

14. Ibid., 1–2.

15. Jean-Louis Comolli, "Machines of the Visible," in *The Cinematic Apparatus,* ed. de Lauretis and Heath, 121–22. See also Comolli, "Technique et idéologie," *Cahiers du cinéma* 229 (May–June 1971): 9–15, translated as "Technique and Ideology: Camera, Perspective, Depth of Field," *Film Reader* 2 (1977): 132–38; "II. Profondeur du champ: la double scène (suite) (Notes pour un histoire materialiste . . . suite)," *Cahiers du cinéma* 231 (August–September 1971): 42–49; and "La profondeur du champ 'primitive'" *Cahiers du cinéma* 233 (November 1971): 40–45, translated as "Technique and Ideology: Camera, Perspective, Depth of Field [parts 3 and 4]," in *Narrative, Apparatus, Ideology,* ed. Philip Rosen (New York: Columbia University Press, 1986), 421–43.

16. Comolli, "Machines of the Visible," 121–22.

17. Ibid., 122.

18. Ibid., 137–38.

19. Ibid., 121–22; Comolli, "Technique and Ideology," 137–38.

20. Comolli, "Technology and Ideology," 132.

21. Heath, "Technology as Historical and Cultural Form," 2.

22. Sigmund Freud, *The Interpretation of Dreams* (New York: Avon, 1965), 574–75; cited in Jean-Louis Baudry, "The Apparatus: Metapsychological Approaches to the Impression of Reality in the Cinema," *Camera Obscura* 1 (Fall 1976): 105.

23. Joan Copjec, "Cinematic Pleasure and Sexual Difference: The Delirium of Clinical Perfection," *Oxford Literary Review* 8 (1986): 57–65. See also Jacqueline Rose, "The Cinematic Apparatus—Problems in Contemporary Theory," in *The Cinematic Apparatus,* ed. de Lauretis and Heath, 172–86, reprinted in Rose, *Sexuality in the Field of Vision* (London: Verso, 1986), 199–213.

24. See Louis and Auguste Lumière, "Sur un procède de tirage de microphotographies des-

tinées à la projection," *Bulletin de la Société Française de Photographie* (1890), 294. See also Auguste Lumière, "Micro-photographie du spirochoete de Schaudinn et Hoffmann," *Société Médicale des Hôpitaux de Lyon* (20 June 1905).

25. Jacob Opper, *Science and the Arts: A Study of Relationships from 1600–1900* (Rutherford, N.J.: Fairleigh Dickinson University Press, 1973), 35.

26. Michel Foucault, *The Order of Things: An Archaeology of the Human Sciences* (New York: Vintage Books, 1973), 129–30.

27. Foucault, *The Order of Things*, 239–40, my emphasis.

28. Ibid., 237.

29. Robert G. Frank, "American Physiologists in German Laboratories, 1865–1914," in Gerald L. Geison, ed., *Physiology in the American Context* (Bethesda, Md.: American Physiological Society, 1987), 14.

30. See Merriley Borell, "Extending the Senses: The Graphic Method," *Medical Heritage* 2, no. 2 (March/April 1986): 114–21, and "Instruments and an Independent Physiology: The Harvard Physiological Laboratory, 1871–1906," in *Physiology in the American Context*, ed. Geison, 293–321. Also see Stanley Joel Reiser, *Medicine and the Reign of Technology* (New York: Cambridge University Press, 1978), 91–122.

31. For an account of physiological optics, see Jonathan Crary, "Techniques of the Observer," *October* 45 (1988): 3–36, a revised version of which appears in his *Techniques of the Observer: On Vision and Modernity in the Nineteenth Century* (Cambridge: MIT Press, 1990), 97–136.

32. See Sander L. Gilman, *Seeing the Insane* (New York: John Wiley and Sons, 1982); Sander L. Gilman, ed., *The Face of Madness: Hugh W. Diamond and the Origin of Psychiatric Photography* (Secaucus, N.J.: Citadel Press, 1976); Alan Sekula, "The Body in the Archive," *October* 39 (1986): 1–64; and John Tagg, *The Burden of Representation: Essays on Photographies and Histories* (Minneapolis: University of Minnesota Press, 1993).

33. Tagg, *The Burden of Representation*, 11.

34. Borell, "Extending the Senses," 46.

35. Christian Metz, *Language and Cinema,* trans. Donna Jean Umiker-Sebeok (The Hague: Mouton, 1974); and *Film Language,* trans. Michael Taylor (New York: Oxford University Press, 1974). Applied over the past two decades in nearly every area of cultural analysis, including some fields of science, semiotics is strikingly absent from studies of physiology (with the exception of Frank's casual reference to physiology's language).

36. Tom Gunning, "'Primitive' Cinema—A Frame Up? or, The Trick's on Us," *Cinema Journal* 28, no. 2 (Winter 1989): 9.

37. Linda Williams, *Hard Core: Power, Pleasure, and the "Frenzy of the Visible"* (Berkeley and Los Angeles: University of California Press, 1989), 52. Williams cites Hendricks, *Origins of the American Film,* 92–93.

38. Films discussed are in the Library of Congress Paper Prints Collection, Washington, D.C. Also relevant to this discussion are many of the physical culture films also held in this collection, including *Physical Culture Lesson* (American Mutoscope and Biograph Company, 1906), *Chest and Neck Development* (Winthrop Press, 1906), and *They Meet on the Mat* (American Mutoscope and Biograph Company, 1902).

2. "Experiments of Destruction"

1. Claude Bernard, *An Introduction to the Study of Experimental Medicine* (New York: Dover Books, 1957), 9.

2. On the role of the elephant in narratives of colonial conquest, see George Orwell's essay "Shooting an Elephant," which describes the plight of a British colonial officer in Burma directed to shoot an elephant who has killed a man (*The Orwell Reader* [New York: Harcourt, Brace and Company, 1956], 3–9). The villagers watch with amusement and disbelief the officer's artless and futile attempts to perform the tricky task of shooting an elephant. Fatimah To-

bing Rony has suggested that the officer's discomfort stems from the reversal of the colonial gaze that takes place in this scene. That his task had become an enactment of a kind of theater of colonial futility is underscored by the remarks of the officer's colleagues later at the club. "Good show," they chide. The technology of electrocution used at Luna Park offers a mastery over the metaphorical colonial drama of conquest, a mastery lacking in the scene Orwell describes (Fatimah Tobing Rony, letter, 15 March 1992).

3. A theme that is not pursued explicitly in this chapter is the issue of the test animal as an identificatory figure. In the chapters that follow, I consider primarily experiments that involve human subjects; most of the experiments considered in chapter 3, however, involve test animals. The material considered below implicitly demonstrates that the animal body functions as a surrogate for the human body in at least two ways. Most obviously, the animal body is substituted for the human body in experiments involving techniques or substances considered too risky to be used on humans. But the test animal is also a stand-in for the human body in a scientific narrative about disciplinary power and corporeal control. The laboratory-as-film-set becomes a microcosmic scene of totalizing optical power and exacting corporeal discipline, a scene of fantasy that allows a degree of technical scrutiny and manipulation of life and death that would be transgressive (if not illegal) were it enacted with human subjects.

4. Nichtenhauser, "A History of Motion Pictures in Medicine" (Bethesda, Md.: National Library of Medicine, History of Medicine Division, circa 1950), 36–38. See also Dr. John Macintyre, "X Ray Records for the Cinematographe," *Archives of Skiagraphy* 1, no. 4 (London: 1897): 37–38; Dr. John Macintyre, "A Demonstration on the X Rays," *Proceedings of the Royal Philosophical Society* 28 (Glasgow, 1897): 267; and Ludwig Braun, *Über Herzbewegung und Herzstoss* (Jena: Denticke, 1898).

5. Macintyre, "X Ray Records," 37.

6. See Stanley Joel Reiser, *Medicine and the Reign of Technology* (Cambridge: Cambridge University Press, 1978); and Merriley Borell, "Extending the Senses: The Graphic Method," *Medical Heritage* 2, no. 2 (March/April 1986): 114–21. The art historian Barbara Maria Stafford proposes a similar model in *Body Criticism: Imaging the Unseen in Enlightenment Art and Criticism* (Cambridge [Mass.] and London: MIT Press, 1991).

7. Jonathan Crary, *Techniques of the Observer: On Vision and Modernity in the Nineteenth Century* (Cambridge: MIT Press, 1990), 2.

8. Some scholars have argued that scientific discourse already included modes of graphic abstraction in earlier periods. For example, Martin J. S. Rudwick analyzes the graphic cross-sectional images making up what he calls the "visual language" of eighteenth- and early-nineteenth-century geology. He points out that geology shared with other natural-history sciences a concern with finding representational forms other than words or mathematical symbols—a project that entailed the development of "ever more abstract, formalized, and theory-laden modes of representation" from the Enlightenment period forward. See Martin J. S. Rudwick, "The Emergence of a Visual Language for Geological Science, 1760–1840," *History of Science* 14 (1976): 151–52.

9. On racial and sexual quantification in nineteenth-century science, see Nancy Leys Stepan, "Race and Gender: The Role of Analogy in Science," *Isis* 77 (1986): 261–77. For an example of this practice, Stepan refers her readers to Paul Topinard, *Anthropology* (London: Chapman and Hall, 1878), part 2, chap. 1–4.

10. Etienne-Jules Marey, *Du mouvement dans les fonctions de la vie* (Paris: Baillière, 1868), 30, translated and quoted in François Dagognet, *Etienne-Jules Marey: A Passion for the Trace* (New York: Zone Books, 1992). Dagognet's pertinent book-length study of Marey's graphic method was published after the completion of this manuscript and hence could not be considered at length in this chapter.

11. See Etienne-Jules Marey, *La méthode graphique dans les sciences expérimentales et particulièrement en physiologie et en médecine* (Paris, 1898), 357–66. On Marey, physiological measurement,

and instrumentation, see Borell, "Extending the Senses," 114–21, and Marta Braun, "The Photographic Work of E. J. Marey," *Studies in Visual Communication* 9, no. 4 (1983): 4–23. It is worth noting that whereas Borell suggests that the physiological recording apparatus *extended* the senses of the observer, Braun suggests that it *substituted* for the senses.

12. Bernard, *An Introduction to the Study of Experimental Medicine,* 8–9.

13. Ibid., 15.

14. Borell, "Extending the Senses," 117.

15. Ibid. My discussion here is indebted to Karl Figlio's suggestion that Bernard's physiology constituted a "technological invasion of life." See Figlio, "The Historiography of Scientific Medicine: An Invitation to the Human Sciences," *Comparative Studies in Society and History* 19, no. 3 (1977): 274–77.

16. Bernard, *An Introduction to the Study of Experimental Medicine,* 9.

17. Dominique François Arago, "Report" (1839), in *Classic Essays on Photography,* ed. Alan Trachtenberg (New Haven: Leete's Island Books, 1980), 21.

18. Arago, *Comptes rendus des séances de L'Académie des sciences* 9, no. 19 (August 1839): 257–66.

19. Borell, "Extending the Senses," 118.

20. Simon Shaffer, "Astronomers Mark Time: Discipline and the Personal Equation," *Science in Context* 2 (1988): 117.

21. Bernard, *An Introduction to the Study of Experimental Medicine,* 16–18.

22. Shaffer, "Astronomers Mark Time," 119.

23. Ibid., 118.

24. Michel Foucault, *Discipline and Punish: The Birth of the Prison* (New York: Random House, 1977), 204.

25. Foucault, *Discipline and Punish,* 204.

26. Arago, "Report," 23 (my emphasis).

27. Further, he assumes that the plate also functions as a reflexive check on the factor of energy absorption and exposure. The element imaged (light or any other form of energy) is also the direct source of the plate's exposure.

28. Comolli, "Technique and Ideology," 136–37.

29. F. A. Talbot, *Moving Pictures: How They Are Made and Worked* (London, 1912; New York: Arno Press, 1970), 20.

30. Steve Neale, *Cinema and Technology: Image, Sound, Color* (Bloomington and Indianapolis: Indiana University Press, 1985), 36.

31. Alan Sekula, "The Body in the Archive," *October* 39 (1986): 13–16.

32. Foucault, *Discipline and Punish,* 155.

33. Foucault, *Discipline and Punish,* 155.

34. See William R. Spriegel and Clark E. Myers, eds., *The Writings of the Gilbreths* (Homewood, Ill: Irwin, 1953), especially 231, 239, 241, and 327–28. See also the compilation film *The Original Films of Frank Gilbreth, 1910–1920,* collection of the Purdue Film Library, West Lafayette, Indiana.

35. In his early writings on film and semiology, Christian Metz argued that movement is what produces the strong impression of reality in the cinema. His argument has interesting implications for a consideration of Marey's rejection of precisely this factor of movement as a rejection of realism, but there is not space to pursue this point here. See *Film Language: A Semiotics of the Cinema,* trans. Michael Taylor (Chicago: University of Chicago Press, 1974), 3–15.

36. Etienne-Jules Marey, *Le mouvement* (Paris: G. Masson, 1894); *Movement,* trans. Eric Pritchard (New York: Appleton Company, 1895).

37. Adolph Nichtenhauser discusses Comandon's work in his unpublished manuscript, "A History of Motion Pictures in Medicine" (Bethesda, Md.: National Library of Medicine, History of Medicine Division, circa 1950). John Maddison, in an entry on scientific film in Roger

Manvell's anthology *Experiment in the Film,* describes Comandon's oeuvre as including X-ray cinematography; microscopic cinematography; and anti–TB films produced during World War I. The microscopic films were the best known, and Maddison describes their complex apparatus, which included a "micro-manipulator," an instrument that scaled down the action of the hand that manipulated the material beneath the microscope's lens in order for the camera to record its activity (John Maddison, "Experiment in the Scientific Film," in *Experiment in the Film,* ed. Roger Manvell (London: Grey Walls Press, 1949), 267.

38. See the very brief account by the surrealist Jacques B. Brunius in Manvell's *Experiment in the Film,* in which it is argued that these films "did much to turn avant-garde toward documentary" (97). This text also makes note of the influence of these films on Jean Painlevé, surrealist and well-known producer of avant-garde and science films in France between the late 1920s and his death in the late 1980s (97). Francisco Aranda, in his briography of Buñuel, makes note of a film program devised for the Sociedad de Cursos y Conferencias in Madrid in early 1927, in which Buñuel included works by Lucien Bull under the title "cinema of the invisible" and "studies in slow motion" alongside René Clair's *Entr'acte* (which was billed as having "several scenes in slow and accelerated motion") and a slow-motion dream sequence from Jean Renoir's *La fille de l'eau* (Francisco Aranda, *Luis Buñuel: A Critical Biography,* trans. David Robinson [London: Secker and Warburg, 1975], 51). I thank Kathy Geritz of the Pacific Film Archive in Berkeley for these references.

39. See Georges Marinesco, "Les troubles de la marche dans l'hémiplegie organique étudies à l'aide du cinématographe," *Semaine médicale* 19 (1899): 225; and Marinesco, "Sur les troubles de la marche dans les paraplegias organiques," *Semaine médicale* 20 (1900): 71.

40. Nichtenhauser, "A History of Motion Pictures in Medicine," 49.

41. See James W. Kernohan's brief biographical sketch of François-Franck in *The Founders of Neurology,* ed. Webb Haymaker (Springfield, Ill.: Charles C. Thomas, 1953), 189–92.

42. Charles Emile François-Franck, *Leçons sur le fonctions motrices du cerveau (réactions volontaires et organiques) et sur l'épilepsie cérébrale* (Paris: Doin, 1887).

43. Foucault, *Discipline and Punish,* 35.

44. François-Franck, "Application de la méthode grapho-photographique à l'étude des réflexes tendineux chez l'homme et chez les animaux," *Comptes rendus de la Société de Biologie* 2 (1904): 9–13. He does not specify the make of his cinema equipment; however, in another publication, he thanks the Lumière brothers and Gaumont (the latter for lights). See also François-Franck, "Technique des prises des vues photo et chrono-photographiques dans l'étude de la mécanique respiratoire des poissons téléosteéns," *Comptes rendus de la Société de Biologie* 58 (1906): 965–67; François-Franck, "Microphotographie en couleur des pièces histologiques avec les plaques autochromes de A. et L. Lumière," *Comptes rendus de la Société de Biologie* 62, no. 1 (1907): 1099–1102; and Louis and Auguste Lumière, "Sur le procédé de tirage de microphotographie destinée à la projection," *Bulletin de la Société française de Photographie,* 1890, 294.

45. Lucien Bull, "La chronophotographie des mouvements rapides," *Travaux de l'Association de l'Institut Marey* 2 (1910): 51. See also Nichtenhauser, "A History of Motion Pictures in Medicine," 51.

3. An Etiology of the Neurological Gaze

1. A small selection of this work includes the anthology *In Dora's Case: Freud, Hysteria, Feminisms,* ed. Charles Bernheimer and Claire Kahane (New York and London: Routledge, 1985); Jacqueline Rose, "Dora—Fragment of an Analysis," originally published in *m/f* 2 (1978): 5–21, and reprinted in Rose, *Sexuality in the Field of Vision* (London: Verso, 1986), 27–47, and in Bernheimer and Kahane, eds., *In Dora's Case,* 128–48; Luce Irigaray, *Speculum de l'autre femme* (Paris: Les Editions de Minuit, 1974), published in English as *Speculum of the Other Woman,* trans. Gillian C. Gill (Ithaca, N.Y.: Cornell University Press, 1985); Georges Didi-Huberman, *Invention de l'hystérie: Charcot et l'iconographie photographique de la Salpêtrière* (Paris: Macula, 1982);

Stephen Heath, "Difference," *Screen* 19, no. 8 (1978/79): 50–112; Leslie Camhi, "Prisoners of Gender," (Ph.D. diss., Yale University, 1991); Yannick Ripa, *La ronde des folles* (Paris: Aubier, 1986), published in English as *Women and Madness: The Incarceration of Women in Nineteenth-Century France,* trans. Catherine du Peloux Menagé (Minneapolis: University of Minnesota Press, 1990); Linda Williams, *Hard Core: Power, Pleasure, and the "Frenzy of the Visible"* (Berkeley and Los Angeles: University of California Press, 1989), especially 46–51; and Lynne Kirby, "Male Hysteria and Early Cinema," *Camera Obscura* 17 (1988): 113–31, reprinted in *Male Trouble,* ed. Constance Penley and Sharon Willis (Minneapolis: University of Minnesota Press, 1993), 67–85.

2. Rose, *Sexuality in the Field of Vision,* 38.

3. Ibid., 96.

4. In *The History of Sexuality,* volume 1, *An Introduction* (New York: Vintage Books, 1980), Foucault stated that it is all very well to denounce psychoanalysis for its normalizing impulse, but psychoanalysis must be credited with freeing the study of mental health and illness from "the political and institutional effects of the perversion-hereditary-degenerescence system"—effects that included eugenics and the racisms of previous scientific regimes (118–19).

5. Michel Foucault, *Power/Knowledge: Selected Interviews and Other Writings, 1972–1977,* ed. Colin Gordon (New York: Pantheon Books, 1977), 60.

6. Rose, *Sexuality in the Field of Vision,* 97; emphasis in original.

7. Gilman, *Seeing the Insane,* 223.

8. See Robert Proctor, *Racial Hygiene: Medicine under the Nazis* (Cambridge [Mass.] and London: Harvard University Press, 1988).

9. See Nancy Leys Stepan, *The Idea of Race in Science: Great Britain, 1800–1960* (London: Macmillan, 1982), especially chapter 1; and "Race and Gender: The Role of Analogy in Science," *Isis* 77 (1986): 261–77.

10. Rose, *Sexuality in the Field of Vision,* 98.

11. The claim of neurobiologist Simon LeVay that he has been able to establish neuro-anatomical evidence of sexual difference in the male brain is a chilling example of this development. Claiming to have experimental proof that the hypothalamus of purportedly gay men is smaller than that of purportedly straight men, LeVay subsequently announced that he would try to show this evidence through magnetic resonance images of the brain (Simon LeVay, "A Difference in Hypothalamic Structure between Heterosexual and Homosexual Men," *Science* 253, no. 5023 [1991]: 1034). For an excellent critical analysis of LeVay's project, see Jennifer Terry, "The Seductive Power of Science in the Making of Deviant Subjectivity," in *The Post Human Body,* ed. Judith Halberstam and Ira Livingston (Bloomington and Indianapolis: Indiana University Press, forthcoming).

12. Foucault, *Power/Knowledge,* 61.

13. See Gilles Deleuze and Félix Guattari, *Anti-Oedipus: Capitalism and Schizophrenia* (New York: Viking Press, 1977).

14. Kaja Silverman, *Male Subjectivity at the Margins* (New York: Routledge, 1992), 187.

15. Silverman, 187.

16. Silverman, 187.

17. Oliver Sacks, *The Man Who Mistook His Wife for a Hat* (New York: Harper Collins, 1987), 93.

18. Chase was trained by the Biograph Company. He shot twenty-five hundred feet of film using their equipment, at a cost of $1,100. References above and following are to the "Twelfth Annual Report to the State Board of Charities, Craig Colony at Sonyea, New York, 1905" and to National Library of Medicine text placards from the exhibition "The Medical Motion Picture" (Bethesda, Md., 1960).

19. Theodore Weisenburg, a professor of neurology at the Philadelphia Medico-Chiurgical College (1906–16) and at the University of Pennsylvania (1918–34), also made cinematic mo-

tion studies of nervous diseases. With the help of the film producer Siegmund Lubin, he began these studies in 1907. His films, which were in distribution through the U.S. Army Medical Museum during World War I, have not been located.

20. See Foucault, *Power/Knowledge*, 151; and *Discipline and Punish: The Birth of the Prison* (New York: Random House, 1979).

21. *Dorland's Illustrated Medical Dictionary* defines epilepsy as a set of "paroxysmal disturbances of brain function that may be manifested as episodic impairment, loss of consciousness, abnormal motor phenomena, psychic or sensory disturbances, or perturbation of the autonomic nervous system." The origin is described as either "idiopathic (cryptogenic, essential, genetic) or symptomatic (acquired, organic)." In other words, modern epilepsy is a heterogeneous and ambiguously genetic or acquired condition. (Elizabeth J. Taylor, ed., *Dorland's Illustrated Medical Dictionary*, 27th ed. [New York: Harcourt Brace Jovanovich, 1988], 568.)

22. "A Long Step Forward: A New Law That Makes for Greater Latitude in the Prosecution of Scientific Work," in Spratling, "Twelfth Annual Report," 29; emphasis in original.

23. "Regarding [his servant] with a gaze that looked forward to her autopsy must have lent life in the Charcot household a macabre tone," remarks Leslie Camhi in "The Servant's Body," an essay forthcoming in *Deviant Bodies,* ed. Jennifer Terry and Jacqueline Urla (Bloomington: Indiana University Press, 1994).

24. Spratling, "Twelfth Annual Report," 33.

25. Walter Greenough Chase, "The Use of the Biograph in Medicine," *Boston Medical and Surgical Journal* 63, no. 2 (1905): 571. See also the accounts in *Motion Picture World,* 23 March 1907.

26. Spratling, "Twelfth Annual Report," 571. Weisenburg provides an account of his own films that is quite similar to that given by Chase: "The superintendent of the colony who kindly placed his material at my disposal selected eighteen of the many hundred epileptics; every one had fits daily, some of them hourly. We placed these patients in the sun with the camera trained on them ready to take a photograph the instance a spasm was manifested, and yet for three hours not a single patient had a sign of a spasm and it was necessary to come the following day before we were able to obtain the photographs. Even under these circumstances, it was difficult to obtain the beginning of epileptic fits" (Theodore Weisenburg, "Moving Picture Illustrations in Medicine," *Journal of the American Medical Association* 59 [28 Dec 1912]: 2310).

27. Theodore Weisenburg, "Moving Picture Illustrations," 2310.

28. Francis X. Dercum, from published discussion following Walter Greenough Chase, "The Use of the Biograph in Medicine," *Transactions of the College of Physicians,* 3d ser., 28 (1906): 16. See also Francis X. Dercum, ed., *A Textbook of Nervous Diseases* (Philadelphia: Lea, 1895).

29. Allan McLane Hamilton, *Railway and Other Accidents with Relation to Injury and Disease of the Nervous System* (New York: William Wood, 1904). For a contemporary analysis of railway trauma and male hysteria, see Kirby, "Male Hysteria and the Early Cinema."

30. Spratling, "Twelfth Annual Report," 33–34.

31. Text placards, "The Medical Motion Picture."

32. Spratling, from published discussion following B. Onuf and Horace LoGrasso, "Researches on the Blood of Epileptics," *Transactions of the Medical Society of the State of New York* 2, nos. 1 and 2 (1905): 272.

33. Ibid., 273.

34. Ibid.; emphasis in original.

35. Ibid.

36. Ibid.

37. Ibid.

38. Spratling, "Description of the Work of the Craig Colony for Epileptics," *Transactions of the College of Physicians,* 3d ser., 28 (1906): 9.

39. Leslie Camhi, from a response to a version of this chapter delivered at the Columbia Seminars for Film and Interdisciplinary Study, the Museum of Modern Art, 19 November 1992.

40. Chase, "The Use of the Biograph in Medicine," 572.

41. Spratling, "Description of the Work of the Craig Colony," 10.

42. Linda Williams, "Film Body: An Implantation of Perversions," in *Narrative, Apparatus, Ideology: A Film Theory Reader,* ed. Philip Rosen (New York: Columbia University Press, 1986), 512.

43. Fulgence Raymond and Pierre Janet, *Névroses et idées fixes* (Paris: Félix Alcan, 1898).

44. On Demenÿ's *portraits vivants,* see Jacques Deslandes, *Histoire comparée du cinéma* (Tournai, Belgium: Casterman, 1966), 159–77.

45. Chase, "The Use of the Biograph in Medicine," 572.

46. Sacks, *The Man Who Mistook His Wife for a Hat,* 93.

47. Lethargic encephalitis also reached epidemic status in other parts of the world between 1915 and 1926.

48. S. Philip Goodhart, M.D., and Benjamin Harris Balser, M.D., Major (M.C.), *Neurological Cinematographic Atlas* (New York: King's Crown Press, 1944).

49. See *Dorland's Illustrated Medical Dictionary,* 27th ed., ed. Taylor, 521.

50. Adolph Nichtenhauser, "A History of Motion Pictures in Medicine" (Bethesda, Md.: National Library of Medicine, History of Medicine Division, circa 1950), 2: 1–23.

51. See Robert Jay Lifton, *The Nazi Doctors: Medical Killing and the Psychology of Genocide* (New York: Basic Books, 1986); and Robert Proctor, *Racial Hygiene: Medicine Under the Nazis* (Cambridge [Mass.] and London: Harvard University Press, 1988).

52. S. P. Goodhart, M.D., and Nathan Savitsky, M.D., "Self-Mutilation in Chronic Encephalitis," *American Journal of the Medical Sciences* 5 (May 1933): 675–76.

53. Goodhart and Savitsky, "Self-Mutilation in Chronic Encephalitis," 677.

54. See John J. Delaney, *Dictionary of Saints* (New York: Doubleday, 1980), 366.

55. Goodhart and Balser, *Neurological Cinematographic Atlas,* 25.

56. Ibid.

57. Karl Abraham, "Manifestations of the Female Castration Complex," *International Journal of Psychoanalysis* 3, no. 1 (March 1922): 13.

4. A Microphysics of the Body

1. Robert Lincoln Watkins, *Diagnosis by Means of the Blood* (New York: The Physicians Book Publishing Co., 1902), 17–18.

2. In *Diagnosis by Means of the Blood,* Watkins cites an article in the *Photogram* of 1897 that credits him with the production of the micro-motoscope (397–98). I have located neither his films nor the *Photogram* essay; however, frame enlargements are reproduced in his book (359, 361). He also states that he demonstrated his instrument to the American Biograph Company, which he claims "intend to go into this line extensively" (367). (Biograph did not.)

3. B. Onuf, M.D., and Horace LoGrasso, M.D., "Researches on the Blood of Epileptics," *Transactions of the Medical Society of the State of New York* 2, nos. 1 and 2 (1905): 263.

4. See, for example, Paul deKruif, *The Microbe Hunters* (New York: Harcourt, Brace and Company, 1926), 3–24.

5. Jonathan Crary, *Techniques of the Observer: On Vision and Modernity in the Nineteenth Century* (Cambridge: MIT Press, 1990).

6. See G. L'E. Turner, "The Microscope as a Technical Frontier in Science," in *Essays on the History of the Microscope* (Oxford: Senecio, 1980), 175–96; and E. M. Nelson, "On the Limits of Resolving Power for the Microscope and Telescope," *Journal of the Royal Microscopical Society,* (October 1906): 521–31.

7. Turner, "The Microscope as a Technical Frontier in Science," 177.

8. C. R. Goring and Andrew Pritchard, *Micrographia: Containing Practical Essays on Reflecting, Solar, Oxy-hydrogen Gas Microscopes; Micrometers, Eyepieces, etc., etc.* (London, 1837). Cited in Turner, "The Microscope as a Technical Frontier in Science," 178.

9. Goring and Pritchard, *Micrographia*, plate II. Reproduced in Turner, "The Microscope as a Technical Frontier in Science," 179.

10. Sir David Brewster, "A Treatise on the Microscope," in *Encyclopaedia Britannica,* 7th ed. (Edinburgh, 1837), 169.

11. *The Penny Cyclopedia for the Diffusion of Useful Knowledge* (London, 1833–43), 5:4; cited in Turner, "The Microscope as a Technical Frontier in Science," 179–80.

12. Turner, "The Microscope as a Technical Frontier in Science," 180–87.

13. On the "cleaning up" of images, see K. Amman and Karen Knorr Cetina, "The Fixation of (Visual) Evidence," in *Representation in Scientific Practice,* ed. Michael Lynch and Steve Woolgar (Cambridge: MIT Press, 1990), 85–121.

14. See Erling Asmussen, "August Krogh—Physiologist," in *Respiratory Adaptations, Capillary Exchange, and Reflex Mechanisms* (proceedings of the August Krogh Centenary Symposium, Srinagar, Kashmir, India, 11–15 October 1974), ed. A. S. Paintal and Pritam Gill-Kumar (Delhi: Vallabhai Patel Chest Institute, University of Delhi, 1977): 1–6. On the relation between physiology and related disciplines such as anatomy and zoology in the United States after 1900, see Diana E. Long, "Physiological Identity of American Sex Researchers Between the Two World Wars," in *Physiology in the American Context,* ed. Gerald L. Geison (Bethesda, Md.: American Physiological Society, 1987), 263–78; see also, in the same volume, Adele E. Clarke, "Research Materials and Reproductive Science in the United States, 1910–1940" (324).

15. Quoted in Asmussen, 3, without reference. The Kroghs note the date as 1909. Their test animal was a rabbit.

16. Quoted in Dora Vallier, "Braque, la peinture et nous," *Cahiers d'art* 29, no. 1 (1954): 16.

17. 269 feet, silent, b/w, National Library of Medicine (Bethesda, Md.), accession no. 0669. Dated 1920 by the National Library of Medicine. See the account of this film in August Krogh and P. Brandt Rehberg, "Kinematographic Methods in the Study of Capillary Circulation," *American Journal of Physiology* 68, no. 2 (1924): 153–60.

18. Michel Foucault, *Discipline and Punish: The Birth of the Prison* (New York: Random House, 1977), 14.

19. August Krogh, *The Anatomy and Physiology of Capillaries* (New Haven: Yale University Press, 1929), 11.

20. Krogh and Rehberg, "Kinematographic Methods in the Study of Capillary Circulation," 153.

21. Ibid., 156.

22. On the importance of the introduction of panchromatic stock to the film industry, see David Bordwell, Janet Staiger, and Kristin Thompson, *The Classical Hollywood Cinema* (New York: Columbia University Press, 1985), 281–97.

23. Clement Greenberg, *Art and Culture: Critical Essays* (Boston: Beacon Press, 1961), 79.

24. See Standish Lawder, *The Cubist Cinema* (New York: New York University Press, 1975).

25. Greenberg, *Art and Culture,* 172.

26. Anthony Michaelis, *Research Films in Biology, Anthropology, Psychology, and Medicine* (New York: Academic Press, 1955), 91–94. He also notes that Imchanitsky of the Marey Institute in 1910 attempted serial section films but had difficulty registering the sections in precisely the same position from frame to frame and did not complete a successful series.

27. John Golding, "Cubism," in *Concepts of Modern Art* (London: Thames and Hudson, 1981), 77.

28. Donna J. Haraway, "A Cyborg Manifesto: Science, Technology, and Socialist-Femi-

nism in the Late Twentieth Century," in *Simians, Cyborgs, and Women: The Reinvention of Nature* (New York: Routledge, 1991), 149.

29. Ibid., 150.

30. W. Bruce Fye, *The Development of American Physiology* (New York and London: Johns Hopkins University Press, 1987), 198.

31. Quoted in *Physiology in the American Context,* ed. Geison, 324.

32. E. R. Clark, J. C. Sandison, and H. C. Hou, "A New Rabbit Board for Use in Studying Living Tissue in Transparent Chambers Introduced into the Ear," *Anatomical Record* 50, no. 2 (August 1931): 171.

33. J. C. Sandison, "A New Method for the Study of Living Growing Tissues by the Introduction of a Transparent Chamber in the Rabbit's Ear," *Anatomical Record* 28, no. 4 (1924): 281. At about the same period, similar studies were done by R. T. Grant, using transillumination of ears from which fur was removed. See C. R. Clark and E. L. Clark, "Observations on Living Arterio-Venous Anastomoses as Seen in Transparent Chambers Introduced into the Rabbit's Ear," *American Journal of Anatomy* 54, no. 2 (March 1934): 231. See also Grant, "Observations on Direct Communications between Arteries and Veins in the Rabbit's Ear," *Heart* 15 (1930): 281; and Grant and E. F. Bland, "Observations on Arterio-Venous Anastomoses in Human Skin and in the Bird's Foot with Special Reference to Reactions to Cold," *Heart* 15 (1931): 385.

34. J. C. Sandison, "The Transparent Chamber of the Rabbit's Ear, Giving a Complete Description of Improved Techniques of Construction and Introduction, and a General Account of Growth and Behavior of Living Cells as Seen with the Microscope," *American Journal of Anatomy* 41, no. 3 (1928): 447–73.

35. In 1930, the Clarks extended their experiment to include an apparatus they called a "preformed tissue chamber." They removed the skin and cartilage of a section of the rabbit ear, covering the exposed blood vessels, nerve supply, and surrounding tissue with a transparent layer of mica. The growth exposed for observation in these chambers was compared with growth that had taken place in the manufactured chambers. However, at no point do the Clarks refer to this "preformed" growth as more natural or normal than the growth taking place in the chambers. The preformed growth is neither model nor control element, but simply another type of normal process, also considered normal.

By 1930, the rabbit's ear had become the site of a broad range of investigations beyond the field of anatomy. The Clarks explain that their chambers "are being used by a number of workers in this department and by several visitors from other departments in the investigation of a variety of problems. These problems included growth of blood and lymphatic capillaries; development, appearance and behavior of cells; transplantation of bone, bone marrow, lymph glands, of kidney and liver tissue; study of the growth of nerves; and reaction of blood vessels to various stimulants and conditions." The window in the rabbit's ear thus became the incongruous site where a variety of research projects coalesced. See E. R. Clark, H. T. Kirby-Smith, R. O. Rex, and R. G. Williams, "Recent Modifications in the Method of Studying Living Cells and Tissues in Transparent Chambers Inserted in the Rabbit's Ear," *Anatomical Record* 47, no. 2 (November 1930): 210.

36. Richard G. Abell and Elliot R. Clark, "A Method of Studying the Effects of Chemicals upon Living Cells and Transparent Chamber Inserted in the Rabbit's Ear," *Anatomical Record* 53, no. 2 (July 1932): 140.

37. E. R. Clark, W. J. Hitschler, H. T. Kirby-Smith, R. O. Rex, and J. H. Smith, "General Observations on the Ingrowth of New Blood Vessels into Standardized Chambers in the Rabbit's Ear, and the Subsequent Changes in the Newly Grown Vessels over a Period of Months," *Anatomical Record* 50, no. 2 (August 1931): 143.

38. Clark and Clark, "Observations on Living Arterio-Venous Anastomoses," 230–31.

39. Copies of Clark films at the National Library of Medicine include *Effect of Heat and Cold on the Circulation of the Blood,* 1933 (no. 0150); *Effects of Massage on the Circulation of the Blood,*

1933 (no. 0534); and *Effect of Massage—Blood Flow before and after Massage—Leucocytes Sticking to Vessel Wall after Massage,* 1933 (no. 1044).

40. This range and mix of techniques is evident throughout Clark and Clark, "Observations on Living Arterio-Venous Anastomoses."

41. Clark, Hitschler, Kirby-Smith, Rex, and Smith, "General Observations on the Ingrowth of New Blood Vessels," 153–54.

42. See Georges Canguilhem, *Le normale et le pathologique* (Paris: Presses Universitaires de France, 1966). Translated by Carolyn R. Fawcett and Robert S. Cohen under the title *The Normal and the Pathological* (New York: Zone Books, 1989).

43. Clark, Hitschler, Kirby-Smith, Rex, and Smith, "General Observations on the Ingrowth of New Blood Vessels," 153–54.

44. Ibid.

45. Michel Foucault, *Power/Knowledge: Selected Interviews and Other Writings, 1972–77* (New York: Pantheon Books, 1980), 81–82.

46. Haraway, "A Cyborg Manifesto," 150–51.

47. Ibid., 180–81.

5. Decomposing the Body

1. Discussion of some of Edison's work follows in the text. In 1907, at the Marey Institute, Carvallo produced X-ray motion pictures of animals using a special double-coated film stock prepared by the Lumière laboratory, where Auguste and Louis had been experimenting with the photographic properties of the X ray since 1896. See Anthony Michaelis, *Research Films in Biology, Anthropology, Psychology, and Medicine* (New York: Academic Press, 1955), 297. On Lumière experiments with X rays, see also Auguste and Louis Lumière, "Recherches photographiques sur le rayons de Röntgen," *Comptes rendus de l'Academie des Sciences* 122 (1896): 382–83. For further detail on Edison and X rays, see Arthur W. Fuchs, "Edison and Roentgenology," *The American Journal of Roentgenology and Radium Therapy* 57, no. 2 (February 1947): 145–56.

2. "Edison and X-Ray Injuries," *Journal of the American Medical Association* 41 (22 August 1903): 499–500.

3. Ruth and Edward Brecher, *The Rays* (Baltimore: Williams and Wilkins, 1969), 163.

4. For an account of scientists' self-sacrificing work with X rays, see Percy Brown, *American Martyrs to Science through the Roentgen Rays* (Springfield, Ill.: Charles C. Thomas, 1936).

5. Charles Warrenne Allen, M.D., "Results in Fifty Cases of Cancer Treated with the Aid of the Roentgen Ray," *New York State Journal of Medicine* 3, no. 7 (1903): 280.

6. Sylvanus P. Thompson, speech to the British Roentgen Society, 5 November 1897, published in *Archives of Skiagraphy* 2 (November 1897); quoted in Otto Glasser, "The Discovery of the Roentgen Rays," in *The Science of Radiology,* ed. Otto Glasser (Springfield, Ill.: Charles C. Thomas, 1933), 2; emphasis in original. As Mark Betz pointed out to me, Thompson was making an allusion to John Milton's *Paradise Lost* and a broader tradition of elite colonial literature in his use of the metaphors of darkness, light, and discovery.

7. Wilhelm Conrad Roentgen, "On a New Kind of Rays," *Science* 3, no. 59 (14 February 1896): 227–31, from the translation in *Nature* by Arthur Stanton from the *Sitzungberichte der Würzburger Physik-medic,* January 1895. A contemporary technical definition might be useful here: X rays are electromagnetic vibrations of short wavelengths produced when electrons moving at high velocities impinge on various substances. Passing a current of high voltage through a vacuum tube, bringing electrons to motion, and then bringing the electrons to a sudden halt by slamming them against a metal target is only one way to generate X rays; the sun is another source. See R. Stuart MacKay, *Medical Images and Displays* (New York: John Wiley, 1984), 16–17.

8. Speculations on the nature of the rays proliferated immediately after Roentgen's experiments, some authors guessing that they were beyond the visible spectrum.

9. Roentgen, "On a New Kind of Rays," 230.

10. This stage illusion is described by Paul Hammond as a precedent to the many skeleton scenarios in the films of Méliès in *Marvelous Méliès* (New York: St. Martin's Press, 1975), 38–40.

11. The physician who made the claim was Dr. William S. Gottheil of New York, and it was reported in published notes on a discussion following a report by Francis P. Kinnicutt, M.D., "Finsen's Phototherapy in Variola and Various Dermatoses," *New York State Journal of Medicine* 3, no. 8 (August 1903): 323.

12. For a comparative study, see Frederick Schavoir, M.D., "Report of Committee on Electric Light Apparatus for Diagnosis and Therapy, and the Roentgen Rays," *Transactions of the American Electro-Therapeutics Association,* publication of the seventh annual meeting (1897): 30–33.

13. Edison's comment was published in *Electrical Engineer,* 19 February 1896. His much-publicized project was initiated by William Randolph Hearst, then publisher of the *New York Journal,* who telegraphed Edison on February 5, 1896, with the message: "WILL YOU AS AN ESPECIAL FAVOR TO THE JOURNAL UNDERTAKE TO MAKE CATHODOGRAPH OF HUMAN BRAIN KINDLY TELEGRAPH ANSWER AT OUR EXPENSE" (Brecher, *The Rays,* 33).

14. See Fuchs, "Edison and Roentgenography," 151–53. Though completely implausible in its time, his science-fiction-like fantasy of using sound to illuminate the brain prefigures the more recent technique of ultrasound imaging.

15. Otto Glasser, *Dr. W. C. Roentgen* (Springfield, Ill.: Charles C. Thomas, 1945), 38.

16. Ibid., 39.

17. "Her Latest Photograph," *The New York Times* (29 May 1898): 14, 61; cited in Stanley Joel Reiser, *Medicine and the Reign of Technology* (New York: Cambridge University Press, 1978), 61.

18. See Sigmund Freud's essay of 1927 on fetishism in *Sexuality and the Psychology of Love,* trans. Philip Reiff (New York: Macmillan, 1963), 214–19.

19. Freud also notes, "In the case of the fetish, too, interest is held up at a certain point— what is possibly the last impression received before the uncanny traumatic one is preserved as fetish" (*Sexuality and the Psychology of Love,* 217). The hand perhaps functions as this point at which interest is arrested, a limit point in popular memory that forestalls knowledge of the violence symbolized in the whole-body X ray.

20. Henry W. Cattell, A.M., M.D., "Roentgen's Discovery—Its Application to Medicine," *The Medical News* 68, no. 7 (15 February 1896): 170. It is interesting to note how many physicians had photosensitive plates on hand.

21. From *Punch,* London, January 25, 1896; quoted in Glasser, "The Discovery of the Roentgen Rays," 9.

22. For an interesting analysis of the fascination with the sexualized concealment of the body see the following two essays on the French psychiatrist G. G. Clérambault's fascination with fabric: Joan Copjec, "The Sartorial Superego," *October* 50 (Fall 1989) 56–95; and Leslie Camhi, "Stealing Femininity: Department Store Kleptomania as Sexual Disorder," *Differences* 5, no. 1 (1993) 26–50.

23. Linda Williams, *Hard Core: Power, Pleasure, and the "Frenzy of the Visible"* (Berkeley and Los Angeles: University of California Press, 1989).

24. Quoted without date in Glasser, "The Discovery of the Roentgen Rays," 8.

25. Other spiritualists of this period seized on all manner of communications technology, including photography and the telephone, to represent extrasensory occurrences and to communicate with the dead. This association between communications technology and the extrasensory finds its more commonplace expression in the nineteenth-century funereal daguerreotype, in which the image functioned to preserve the visage of the newly dead body. The

funereal daguerreotype fixes an image of the body before it decomposes and is buried out of sight.

The X ray also appears in futurist and surrealist art. See Linda Dalrymple Henderson, "Boccioni and the X-Ray: The Quest for Invisible Reality in Early Modern Art," lecture, Metropolitan Museum of Art, 2 October 1988; and "Italian Futurism and the Fourth Dimension," *Art Journal* 41, no. 4 (Winter 1981): 317–23. See also Nancy Allen's essay on medical futurism in *Imagining Tomorrow: History, Technology, and the American Future,* ed. Joseph J. Corn (Cambridge: MIT Press, 1986).

26. Thomas Mann, *The Magic Mountain* (New York: Vintage Books, 1955), 213.

27. Ibid., 215.

28. Ibid., 214.

29. Ibid., 215.

30. Howard Burhans Besemer, M.D., "Septicemia and Death Following X-Ray Burns," *New York State Journal of Medicine* 3, no. 7 (1903): 296–97.

31. Elihu Thomson, "The Rontgen Ray and Its Relation to Physics: A Topical Discussion," *Transactions of the American Institute of Electrical Engineering* 13 (1896): 403-32.

32. Emil H. Grubbé, *X-Ray Treatment: Its Origin, Birth and Early History* (St. Paul and Minneapolis: The Bruce Publishing Company, 1949).

33. Ibid., 79–89.

34. Ibid., 89.

35. Dr. Sinclair Tousey, "Some Radiographs of Obscure Stomach and Intestinal Cases . . . ," *New York Medical Journal* (16 August 1913): 349.

36. J. Kramer Hudson, "Roentgen-Ray Dosimetry," in *The Science of Radiology,* ed. Glasser, 120–38.

37. Michaelis, *Research Films in Biology, Anthropology, Psychology, and Medicine,* 301.

38. See the discussion of figure 1.2 above.

39. See Lewis Gregory Cole, "Gastric Motor Phenomena Demonstrated with the Projecting Kinetoscope," *American Quarterly of Roentgenology* 3, no.1 (1912); and "The Complex Motor Phenomena of Various Types of Unobstructed Gastric Peristalsis," *Archives of the Roentgen Ray* 16 (1911): 242–47.

40. Investigation of contrast media for study of the respiratory, gastrointestinal, and circulatory systems and the urinary tract was begun in 1896 with experiments such as those of Wolf Becher of Berlin, who studied the digestive tracts of animals to whom he had fed food laced with metal salts. For reprints and translations of key texts in the development of contrast media, see *Classic Description in Diagnostic Roentgenology,* vol. 2, ed. André J. Bruwer (Springfield, Ill.: Charles C. Thomas, 1964), 1431–1517, 1605–1728, and 1774–90.

41. Discovery of the nature of the circulatory system was at the core of William Harvey's foundational work in physiology. See Merriley Borell, "Extending the Senses: The Graphic Method," *Medical Heritage* 2, no. 2 (March/April 1986): 114. See also chapter 1 above.

42. Sigmund Freud, *Inhibitions, Symptoms, and Anxiety* (London: Hogarth Press, 1948), 130–42.

43. Ibid., 137.

44. See Bruwer (ed.), *Classic Description in Diagnostic Roentgenology,* vol. 2, 1275. According to Janker's voice-over narration, the 1932 film is no longer available except as reproduced in the 1962 film. The English translation of the title of the 1962 film is *Development and Present State of Cineradiography* (produced at the Strahlenklinik Janker, Bonn, 35 minutes, b/w, sound; available in the University of Rochester School of Medicine and Dentistry, Department of Radiology Teaching Film Collection, University of Rochester School of Medicine and Dentistry, currently undergoing preservation at the National Library of Medicine, Bethesda, Maryland).

45. For an interesting account of Warren's early experiments, see George H. S. Ramsey, M.D., "Cinefluorography at the University of Rochester School of Medicine and Dentistry," in

Cinefluorography, Proceedings of the First Annual Symposium on Cinefluorography, University of Rochester School of Medicine and Dentistry, Rochester, New York (Springfield, Ill.: Charles C. Thomas, 1960), 121–28. News of Warren's role in the plutonium experiments was made public during the final revisions of my manuscript. See Corydon Ireland, "Plutonium Injections Leave Legacy of Anger," *Rochester Democrat and Chronicle,* 3 January 1994, 1A, 8A.

46. On the avant-garde films of Watson and Webber, see Lisa Cartwright, "Literary Modernism and the Emergence of 'the Right Wing of Film Art': The Films of James Sibley Watson, Jr., and Melville Folsom Webber," in *Lovers of Cinema: The Early American Film Avant-Garde,* ed. Jan-Christopher Horak (Madison: University of Wisconsin Press, forthcoming).

47. See Harry L. Segal, M.D., and James S. Watson, Jr., M.D., "Color Photography through the Flexible Gastroscope," *Gastroenterology* 10, no. 4 (April 1948): 575–85. See also Watson, Segal, and Sydney A. Weinberg, "Gastroscopic Color Photography," *Journal of the Biological Photographers' Association* 16, no. 1 (September 1947): 23–28. Watson and Segal cite as their precedents the attempt by Lange and Meltzung in 1898 to photograph the interior wall of the stomach by introducing a camera attached to a rubber tube.

48. Edgar Allan Poe, "The Fall of the House of Usher," in *The Portable Poe,* ed. Philip Van Doren Stern (New York: Viking Books, 1945), 257.

49. Watson, Dr. Sydney Weinberg (who was also a sculptor), and Dr. Raymond Gramiak were responsible for this development. See "Audiovisual News," *Journal of Medical Education* 28, no. 3 (March 1953): 77. Comandon and Lomon produced one of the earliest X-ray motion pictures of the human heart in 1924.

50. Robert Proctor, *Racial Hygiene: Medicine under the Nazis* (Cambridge [Mass.] and London: Harvard University Press, 1988), 163. He quotes from Chantraine's essay, "Naturwissenschaft und Raumsichtigkeit," *Ziel und Weg* 6 (1936): 7.

51. Both films are by U.S. director Jack Arnold, released in 1954 and 1953, respectively. See James Cameron, *Three Dimensional Movies and Expanded Screen* (Coral Gables, Fla.: Cameron Publishing Co., 1953); R. M. Yahes, *3D Movies* (Jefferson, N.C.: McFarland & Co., 1989); and Lenny Lipton, *Foundations of the Stereoscopic Cinema* (New York: Van Nostrand and Reinhold Co., 1982).

52. The Watson 3-D technique entailed moving the subject and the X-ray source synchronously before a single static camera. Two prints of the same 70 millimeter film were synchronously projected through polarized filters and viewed through polarized glasses. The equipment is now in the collection of the George Eastman House International Museum of Photography and Film in Rochester, New York.

53. See J. Jacobi, R. Janker, and W. Schmitz. "Investigation with Simultaneously Taken Electrocardiographs, X-Ray Motion Pictures, and Ionographs" (1931), translated in Bruwer (ed.), *Classic Description in Diagnostic Roentgenology,* 2: 1277–78.

6. Women and the Public Culture of Radiography

1. See Diana Phillips Mahoney, "Picture This," *Computer Graphics World,* September 1992, 43–52; the *New England Journal of Medicine*'s monthly one-page special section on medical imaging, begun in March 1992; the *Journal of Reproductive Medicine*'s January 1992 special issue, "Imaging Techniques in Reproductive Medicine"; *National Geographic*'s January 1987 feature photo-essay by Howard Sochurek, "Medicine's New Vision"; and the notorious 30 April 1965 and August 1990 issues of *Life* magazine that feature Leonard Nilsson's images of the fetus in utero.

2. On the recent controversy over federal funding of breast cancer research in the military, see Susan Love's commentary, "Breast Cancer: What the Military Should Do with Its $210 Million," *Journal of the American Medical Association* 269, no. 18 (1993): 2417; Eliot Marshall, "The Politics of Breast Cancer," *Science* 259 (1993): 616; and Eliot Marshall, "Breast Cancer's Forced March?" *Science* 258 (1992): 732–34.

3. As, for example, in the Tailhook incident, publicized in 1993.

4. Love, "Breast Cancer," 2417. See also the hotly debated Canadian study suggesting that mammography does not benefit women younger than fifty. A. B. Miller et al., "Canadian Breast Cancer Screening Study 1: Breast Cancer and Death Rate Among Women Aged 40 to 49 Years," *Canadian Medical Association Journal* 147 (1992): 1459–76.

5. Lisa Belkin, "Top TB Peril: Not Taking the Medicine," *The New York Times,* 18 November 1991, B1.

6. Elizabeth Holtzman, comptroller, "Poverty and Breast Cancer in New York City," City of New York, Office of the Comptroller, Office of Policy Management, October 1990. This report is also discussed in Elisa Solomon, "The Politics of Breast Cancer," *Camera Obscura* 28 (1992): 162.

7. Elizabeth Holtzman, comptroller, "Radiation out of Control: The Department of Health's Bureau for Radiation Control Is Not Inspecting All X-Ray Equipment in New York City," City of New York, Office of the Comptroller, January 1992. That the problem is not simply one of access is made clear in a 1985 report of the federal Food and Drug Administration, which states that 36 percent of mammography facilities tested produced images of unacceptable quality. This study, not released to the public until 1990, provoked the American College of Radiology (the main national professional body of radiologists) to institute a mammography accreditation program in 1986. For an account of the FDA document and a description of the ACR program, see "HRG Report on Screening Mammography: Part 2," *Public Citizen Health Research Group Health Letter* 7, no. 2 (September 1991): 1–6.

8. Breast cancer may occur in men, but only rarely. Susan Love states that breast cancer accounts for less than 1 percent of male malignancies (Susan Love, M.D., with Karen Lindsey, *Dr. Susan Love's Breast Book* [Reading, Mass.: Addison Wesley, 1990], 276–77).

9. For a discussion of more recent representations of women in discourses surrounding epidemic illness, see Paula A. Treichler, "Beyond *Cosmo*: AIDS, Identity, and Inscriptions of Gender," *Camera Obscura* 28 (1992): 21–77.

10. Desmond Callan, in a letter to the editor, "Declining Living Standards Account for Sharp Rise in TB Cases," *The New York Times,* 17 May 1992, sec. 4, 16. By 1960 the National Tuberculosis Association, confident that the decline in incidence would continue, eliminated the disease from its title altogether to become the American Lung Association. Treatment drugs included streptomycin, a drug first successfully tested on people with TB in 1944, and isoniazid, a drug known to physicians since 1912 but not tested by commercial laboratories for use as a TB treatment until 1951—that is, after the proven commercial viability of streptomycin.

11. In some states, surveillance and control mechanisms ranged from the relatively innocuous to the blatantly violating (such as the removal of children from homes of tubercular parents, or the making mandatory of TB case reporting). See Royal Ford, "30 Years Apart, Siblings United Again in Maine," *Boston Globe,* 18 March 1990, 3; and Daniel Fox, "Social Policy and City Politics: Tuberculosis Reporting in New York 1899–1900," *Bulletin of the History of Medicine* 49 (1975): 169–95. For a sense of more recent surveillance mechanisms, see J. Busby, "Texas Department of Health Will Seek Mandatory TB Screening in Jails," *Texas Medicine* 87, no. 2 (February 1991): 52–53.

12. J. A. Jereb et al., "Tuberculosis Morbidity in the United States: Final Data, 1990," *Morbidity and Mortality Weekly Report: Centers for Disease Control Surveillance Summaries* 40, no. 3 (1991): 23–27.

13. Peter Davis and John McKinlay, "Society, Not Science, Has Failed TB," *The New York Times,* 3 November 1992, A18. The authors of this letter to the editor are health policy researchers.

14. William Osler, "The Home and Its Relation to the Tuberculosis Problem," *Medical News* 83 (1903): 1105–6; cited in Barbara Bates, *Bargaining for Life: A Social History of Tuberculo-*

sis (Philadelphia: University of Pennsylvania Press, 1992), 234. On the targeting of women for TB nursing, see especially chapters 11 and 13.

15. Bates, *Bargaining for Life,* 234.

16. Edward H. Beardsley, "Race as a Factor in Health," in *Women, Health, and Medicine in America,* ed. Rima D. Apple (New Brunswick, N.J.: Rutgers University Press, 1990), 126.

17. A 1939 text, *Primitive Tuberculosis,* states that "the disease is a veritable scourge" in the African American community, and that the death rate was more than twice as high among insured blacks than among insured whites, and eleven times higher among black boys than among white boys of the same age (S. Lyle Cummins, *Primitive Tuberculosis* [London: John Bale Publications, 1939], 97). The data are taken from a Metropolitan Life Insurance Company report of 1920. This outrageously titled book is a racist construction of TB's genetic lineage among peoples of Africa and India, a lineage in which the author includes African Americans, Native Americans, and animals. Unfortunately, many statistics from this period are couched in such racist arguments.

18. The surveillance of the interior of the body through the X ray was only one component of the struggle to bring tuberculosis under control. The census bureau and other organizations used a whole battery of techniques to manage TB, many of which are chronicled in the 1939 public health film *On the Firing Line* (a print of which is in the collection of the National Library of Medicine).

19. On the inscription of the body's interior in medical discourse from the eighteenth to the early nineteenth century, see Michel Foucault, *The Birth of the Clinic: An Archaeology of Medical Perception* (New York: Random House, 1973), especially chapters 7–9; and Barbara Maria Stafford, *Body Criticism: Imaging the Unseen in Enlightenment Art and Medicine* (Cambridge [Mass.] and London: MIT Press, 1991).

20. F. M. McPhedran, "Diagnosis and Classification of Pulmonary Tuberculosis in Childhood and Adolescence," *American Review of Tuberculosis* 20 (1929): 532–636.

21. I deal with this issue in its historical context at length in chapter 5.

22. Anne Friedberg, "A Denial of Difference: Theories of Cinematic Identification," in *Psychoanalysis and Cinema,* ed. E. Anne Kaplan (New York: Routledge, 1990), 41–42. Recent work by Allucquere Roseanne Stone suggests that identification with machines is indeed possible. See Allucquere Roseanne Stone, "Will the Real Body Please Stand Up?: Boundary Stories about Virtual Cultures," in *Cyberspace: First Steps,* ed. Michael Benedict (Cambridge: MIT Press, 1991).

23. Because these scenes were shot from a fluoroscopic screen, exposure levels were much lower than they would have been had the scenes been shot in the direct method.

24. For recent discussions of these statistics and their interpretation, see "Breast Cancer Research: A Special Report," ed. Eliot Marshall, *Science* 259 (January 1993): 617–38.

25. Albert Salomon, "Contributions to the Pathology and Clinical Picture of Carcinoma of the Breast," *Archiv für klinische Chirurgie* 101 (1913): 573–68, as cited in Ronald L. Eisenberg, *Radiology: An Illustrated History* (St. Louis: Mosby-Year Book, Inc., 1992), 364.

26. Eisenberg, *Radiology: An Illustrated History,* 364.

27. Helen Ingleby and Jacob Gershon-Cohen, *Comparative Anatomy, Pathology, and Roentgenology of the Breast* (Philadelphia: University of Pennsylvania Press, 1960), xvii.

28. V. Kremens, "Roentgenology of the Breast," *American Journal of Roentgenology* 80 (1958): 1005.

29. For an account of this work, see Eisenberg, *Radiology: An Illustrated History,* 366.

30. Interestingly, Dr. Susan Love states that she has trouble with the idea of a baseline mammogram for precisely these reasons. She suggests that serial mammograms are a more important indicator because they provide a view of change over time, rather than a gauge of aberrance from a supposed norm (*Dr. Susan Love's Breast Book,* 180).

31. J. Gershon-Cohen and Albert Strickler, "Roentgenologic Examination of the Normal Breast," *American Journal of Roentgenology* 40, no. 2 (1930): 189–201.

32. Rosalind Pollack Petchesky, "Foetal Images: The Power of Visual Culture in the Politics of Reproduction," in *Reproductive Technologies: Gender, Motherhood, and Medicine,* ed. Michelle Stanworth (Minneapolis: University of Minnesota Press, 1987), 69. On the public culture of obstetrical ultrasound, see also Janelle Sue Taylor, "The Public Fetus and the Family Car: From Abortion Politics to a Volvo Advertisement," *Public Culture* 4, no. 2 (Spring 1992): 67–80; and Carol Stabile, "Shooting the Mother: Fetal Photography and the Photography of Disappearance," *Camera Obscura* 28 (1992): 179–205.

33. See Edward Yoxen's thorough account of ultrasound's early history, "Seeing with Sound: A Study of the Development of Medical Images," in *The Social Construction of Technological Systems,* ed. Wiebe E. Bijker, Thomas P. Hughes, and Trevor Pinch (Cambridge: MIT Press, 1989), 281–306. Here I draw from pages 283–84.

34. In this paragraph, my source is Yoxen, "Seeing with Sound," 284–89.

35. Lyle A. French, John J. Wild, and Donald Neal, "Attempts to Determine Harmful Effects of Pulsed Ultrasonic Vibrations," *Cancer* 4, no. 2 (March 1951): 342–44.

36. French et al., 342–3. The source they cite is C. W. Porter, "Curious Effects of Ultrasound," *California Engineer,* April 1939.

37. J. J. Wild and Donald Neal, "Use of High-Frequency Ultrasonic Waves for Detecting Changes of Texture in Living Tissue," *Lancet* (24 March 1951): 655–57.

38. John J. Wild and John M. Reid, "Further Pilot Echographic Studies on the Histologic Structures of Tumors of the Living Intact Human Breast," *American Journal of Pathology* 28, no. 2 (1952): 843, my emphasis.

39. Ibid., 839.

40. Ibid., 656.

41. Ibid., 845.

42. For a decade-by-decade account of ultrasound mammography research, see Elizabeth Kelly-Fry, "Influences on the Development of Ultrasound Pulse-Echo Breast Instrumentation in the United States," in *Ultrasound Mammography,* ed. Pat Harper (Baltimore: University Park Press, 1985), 1–20.

43. Ibid., 3.

44. Ibid., 2.

45. For more on these techniques, see Barbara Monsees, "Thermography, Transillumination, Light Scanning, and Magnetic Resonance Imaging," in the charmingly titled *The Female Breast and Its Disorders,* ed. George W. Mitchell Jr. and Lawrence W. Bassett (Baltimore: Williams and Wilkins, 1990), 161–71.

46. For a recent summary of the history of mammography see Richard A. Cooper, "Mammography," in *Textbook of Breast Diseases,* ed. John H. Isaacs (St. Louis: Mosby-Year Book, Inc., 1992), 47–86.

47. See Carol A. Brown, "Women Workers in the Health Services Industry," in *Women and Health: The Politics of Sex in Medicine,* ed. Elizabeth Fee (Farmingdale, N.Y.: Baywood Press, 1983), 105–16.

48. Medicare coverage for mammography began in 1991.

49. This project is under way in the activities of groups like the National Breast Cancer Coalition and the Women's Health Action and Mobilization and in activist video projects like Ngozi Onwurah's 1991 *The Body Beautiful* (a film about the body, beauty, and pleasure in the context of a mother/daughter relationship in which the mother has undergone a mastectomy and lives with rheumatoid arthritis) and Kathy High's interventionist history of reproductive politics, *Underexposed: The Temple of the Fetus* (1993).

Index

Abraham, Karl, 78-79
acromegaly, 41
ACT-UP (AIDS Coalition to Unleash
    Power), 169
activism, 144-45, 169-70
agency, xiv, 152; of the experimental appara-
    tus, 43, 85-86, 89, 128; of the test sub-
    ject/object, 42, 48, 54, 80, 87-88, 92-93,
    128, 163-64; of women, 108-9, 146,
    153, 169-70
AIDS, 148, 169, 170
alcoholism, 66, 70
Allen, Nancy, 184 n. 25
American Mutoscope and Biograph Com-
    pany, 56-57; *Female Facial Expressions,* 14;
    Photographing a Female Crook, 14. *See also*
    epilepsy biographs
amputation, 110, 127, 128
anatomy, xiii, 11, 26, 67, 98; pathological,
    xiii, 11, 47, 51, 55, 162, 165
angiography, infant, 132, 133, 136, 137, 139
animal: as surrogate for human, 42-44, 134-
    36, 174 n. 3; as test subject, 20-22, 24-
    26, 38-39, 42-44, 91-95, 98-105, 131,
    134-36, 137; X-ray experiments on, 131, 134-
    36, 137
Another to Conquer, 149
anthropology, xvii, 12
anthropometry, 51
anxiety, xiv, 18; cultural, 4, 18, 117-21; and
    repetition, 132-33; scientific, 4, 6, 39,
    61, 63, 73-79, 84-87, 93, 162
Arago, Dominique François, 29-30, 32, 110,
    129. *See also* daguerrotype
Arnold, Jack, 185 n. 51

*Arrivée d'un train en gare de Villefranche-sur-
    Saône,* 2;
art, 91, 108; high art, 107, 108, 138-39, 140;
    Jewish, 141; modernist, xiii, xiv, 91, 92,
    95, 96, 97, 108, 137-39, 141
astronomy, 30-31, 32, 43, 87. *See also* body,
    astral; observation, astronomical
athetosis, 67
autopsy, xiii, 10, 24, 37, 57-58, 64, 126

bacteriology, xiii
Balser, Benjamin Harris, 72-78
barium, 131, 157
Bates, Barbara, 149
Baudry, Jean-Louis, 5-8, 10
Beardsley, Edward H., 149
behavior, 51-54. *See also* perversion
Bell, Alexander Graham, 71
Bernard, Claude, 11, 17-20, 26-28, 31, 36,
    39, 46, 60, 126, 132
Bertillon, Alphonse, 35
Besant, Annie, 119, 121
Bichat, Marie-François-Xavier, 11
bioengineering, 82
biologism, 50, 74, 149
biology, xi, xiii, 1, 9-10, 13, 104, 149
biomedicine, xiii
biopsy, 160, 165, 167
birth, 132
birth trauma, 132-33
bismuth, 131
blood, 140; circulation of, 65, 90-92, 93-95,
    100-103, 131-32; invasive experimenta-
    tion on vessels, 27, 93-95, 99, 100-103,
    105, 130, 181 n. 35; as site of pathology,

189

Lisa Cartwright is an assistant professor of English and visual and cultural studies at the University of Rochester. With Paula A. Treichler, she is coeditor of *Imaging Technologies, Inscribing Science,* a forthcoming anthology on gender and the visual and inscriptive cultures of medicine and science.